MW00776373

PERSONAL FITNESS

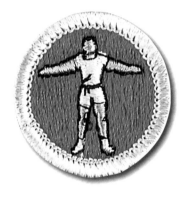

PRIBULA

BOY SCOUTS OF AMERICA®

Requirements

Note: If meeting any of the requirements for this merit badge is against the Scout's religious convictions, the requirement does not have to be done if the Scout's parents and the proper religious advisers state in writing that to do so would be against religious convictions. The Scout's parents must also accept full responsibility for anything that might happen because of this exemption.

1. Do the following:

   a. Before completing requirements 2 through 9, have your health-care practitioner give you a physical examination, using the Scout medical examination form. Describe the examination. Tell what questions the doctor asked about your health. Tell what health or medical recommendations the doctor made and report what you have done in response to the recommendations. Explain the following:

      (1) Why physical exams are important

      (2) Why preventive habits are important in maintaining good health

      (3) Diseases that can be prevented and how

      (4) The seven warning signs of cancer

      (5) The youth risk factors that affect cardiovascular fitness in adulthood

   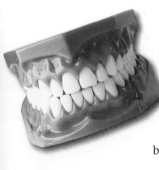

   b. Have a dental examination. Get a statement saying that your teeth have been checked and cared for. Tell how to care for your teeth.

35927
ISBN 978-0-8395-3286-6
©2006 Boy Scouts of America
2008 Printing

2. Explain to your merit badge counselor verbally or in writing what personal fitness means to you, including

   a. Components of personal fitness.

   b. Reasons for being fit in all components.

   c. What it means to be mentally healthy.

   d. What it means to be physically healthy and fit.

   e. What it means to be socially healthy. Discuss your activity in the areas of healthy social fitness.

   f. What you can do to prevent social, emotional, or mental problems.

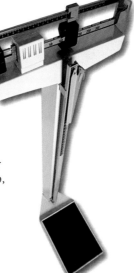

3. With your counselor, answer and discuss the following questions:

   a. Are you free from all curable diseases? Are you living in such a way that your risk of preventable diseases is minimized?

   b. Are you immunized and vaccinated according to the advice of your health-care provider?

   c. Do you understand the meaning of a nutritious diet and know why it is important for you? Does your diet include foods from all food groups?

   d. Are your body weight and composition what you would like them to be, and do you know how to modify them safely through exercise, diet, and behavior modification?

   e. Do you carry out daily activities without noticeable effort? Do you have extra energy for other activities?

   f. Are you free from habits relating to poor nutrition and the use of alcohol, tobacco, drugs, and other practices that could be harmful to your health?

   g. Do you participate in a regular exercise program or recreational activities?

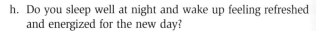

h. Do you sleep well at night and wake up feeling refreshed and energized for the new day?

i. Are you actively involved in the religious organization of your choice, and do you participate in its youth activities?

j. Do you spend quality time with your family and friends in social and recreational activities?

k. Do you support family activities and efforts to maintain a good home life?

4. Explain the following about physical fitness:

a. The components of physical fitness

b. Your weakest and strongest component of physical fitness

c. The need to have a balance in all four components of physical fitness

d. How the components of personal fitness relate to the Scout Law and Scout Oath

5. Explain the following about nutrition:

a. The importance of good nutrition

b. What good nutrition means to you

c. How good nutrition is related to the other components of personal fitness

d. The three components of a sound weight (fat) control program

6. Before doing requirements 7 and 8, complete the aerobic fitness, muscular strength, flexibility, and body composition tests as described in the *Personal Fitness* merit badge pamphlet. Record your results and identify those areas where you feel you need to improve.

7. Outline a comprehensive 12-week physical fitness program using the results of your fitness tests. Be sure your program incorporates the endurance, intensity, and warm-up guidelines discussed in the *Personal Fitness* merit badge pamphlet. Before beginning your exercises, have the program approved by your counselor and parents.

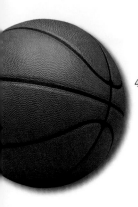

8. Complete the physical fitness program you outlined in requirement 7. Keep a log of your fitness program activity (how long you exercised; how far you ran, swam, or biked; how many exercise repetitions you completed; your exercise heart rate; etc.). Repeat the aerobic fitness, muscular strength, and flexibility tests every two weeks and record your results. After the 12th week repeat all four tests, record your results, and show improvement in each one. Compare and analyze your preprogram and postprogram body composition measurements. Discuss the meaning and benefit of your experience, and describe your long-term plans regarding your personal fitness.

9. Find out about three career opportunities in personal fitness. Pick one and find out the education, training, and experience required for this profession. Discuss what you learned with your counselor, and explain why this profession might interest you.

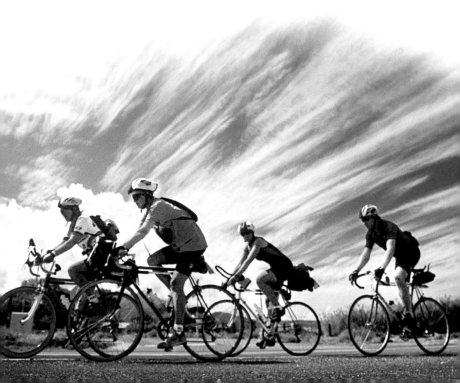

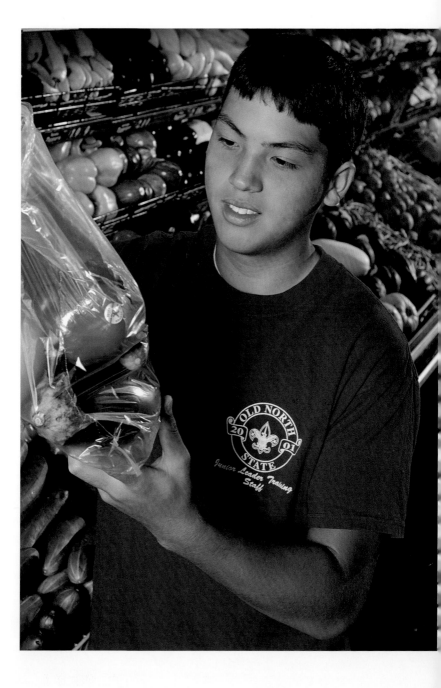

Contents

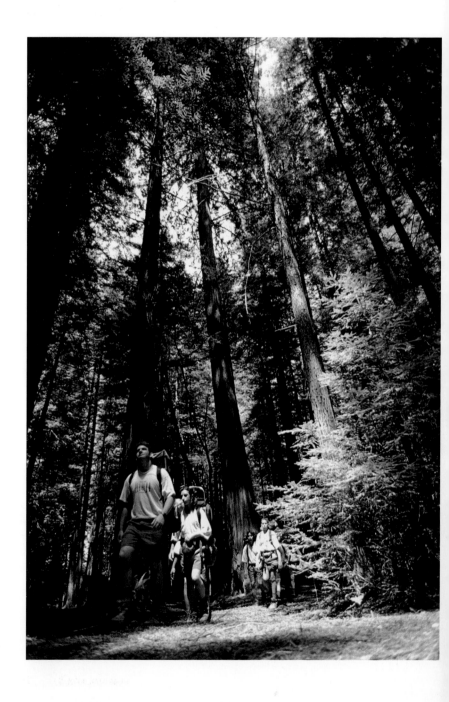

Strive for a New Level of Personal Fitness

Regardless of your current level of personal fitness, in the 12 weeks it will take you to complete the athletic requirements for this merit badge, you will be in better shape, feel better about yourself, have more energy, and gain self-confidence in your overall abilities.

Fitness is the capacity to achieve the best quality of life possible. *Personal fitness* is your individual effort and desire to be the best you can be. If you are *fit,* you are healthy.

To reach your goal, think about how your body works in various situations and about the things that affect your quality of life. Personal fitness is not just physical.

> There are many different elements that make up personal fitness. These elements involve your:
>
> - Mind—mental willpower and alertness, emotional balance, and social skills
> - Body—physical health, nutrition, and athletic fitness
> - Spirit—faith, core values, how you take care of yourself and reach out to help others
>
> It is important to strengthen each element of your personal fitness because each element affects the total person you are and your development and well-being.

All elements of personal fitness work together, interacting and influencing one another. If you are strong in body but weak in spirit, your overall level of personal fitness will drop. Just as a high level of fitness in one area will boost another area, a low level of fitness in one element will limit your accomplishments in the other elements.

Think of a bridge your troop lashes together with ropes. How strong would that bridge be if some of the poles or boards were rotted, or if some of the knots were loose? The bridge would be only as strong as its weakest lashing or rotted post. If we replace the rotted boards and poles and tighten the lashings, the bridge will be much stronger. Think of your personal fitness in the same way. By replacing bad habits with good ones and reinforcing our overall health in simple but surefire ways, our quality of life can dramatically improve, putting us on better footing in every aspect of our lives.

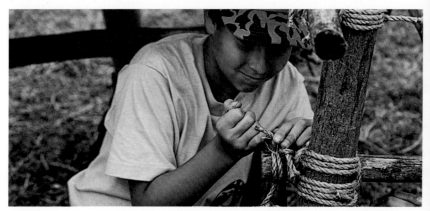

A bridge is only as strong as its weakest element, just like your personal fitness.

Rate Your Own Personal Fitness

In earning this merit badge, you will learn how to evaluate your personal fitness level and begin an exercise program for improvement.

You will need to rate yourself as far as your personal fitness. Objectively rating one's social, mental, emotional, and spiritual status is not easy. In earning this merit badge, you will learn to evaluate your physical fitness level and begin an exercise program that you can use for the rest of your life.

You might never have thought about your level of personal fitness. You may go from day to day taking part in activities without appreciating the benefits of a healthy body. Do not take personal fitness for granted!

Having a healthy level of fitness means that your body is in such good condition that you feel energetic and look healthy. It also means you have the confidence, energy, and endurance to enjoy yourself. And this is the very best time, during your preteen and teen years, to set a lifestyle pattern that will help you stay fit throughout your life.

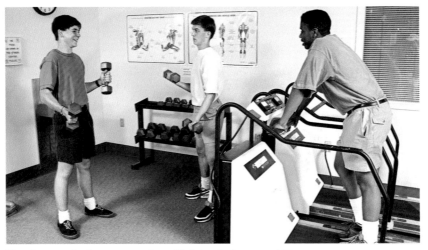

Regular exercise is necessary for a high level of personal fitness.

For example, your personal fitness program must be well-balanced. If you eat properly but do not exercise regularly, you will not be able to perform well in physical activities. Likewise, if you exercise regularly but do not eat well, you may be much more easily tired out and get sick more often. If you are highly active all day at Scout camp but do not prepare a nourishing meal or sleep enough hours that night, you will probably be dragging behind on the next day's hike.

If you become as fit as you can be, your confidence in yourself will grow because you will know that you are making the best possible use of your physical characteristics and makeup. Fill your days with study, sports, and family, troop, or other social activities. Do not fritter away your days with lots of idle time. If you exercise, eat balanced meals, and get enough sleep, you will discover that you have boundless energy to carry you through day-to-day living, as well as any emergencies that arise.

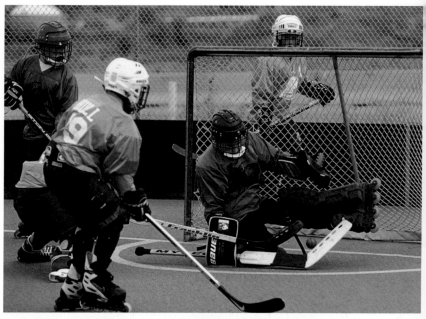

Playing sports with friends will boost your level of personal fitness.

Being personally fit can also help you fulfill the responsibilities of being a Scout. A Scout is cheerful, strong, mentally awake, helpful, and prepared, and does a Good Turn daily. Think about it. It is hard to be prepared for any situation without an excellent level of personal fitness. And having a high level of social fitness will enable you to be kind, courteous, and helpful.

Signs of Poor Personal Fitness

1. Obesity and poor muscle tone

2. Persistent fatigue

3. Often feeling pressured, tense, stressed out

4. Frequent colds, flu, headaches, aches and pains, skin disorders

5. Depression, anxiety, sleeplessness

Your Personal Fitness Test

To begin an evaluation of your personal fitness, ask yourself these questions:

1. Are you free from all curable diseases? Are you living in such a way that your risk of preventable diseases is minimized?

2. Are you immunized and vaccinated according to the advice of your health-care provider?

3. Do you understand the meaning of a nutritious diet and know why it is important for you? Does your diet include foods from all food groups? Do you moderate your intake of high-fat and high-calorie foods?

4. Are your body weight and composition what you would like them to be? Do you know how to modify them safely through exercise, diet, and lifestyle?

5. Do you carry out daily activities without noticeable effort? Do you have extra energy for other activities?

6. Are you free from alcohol, tobacco, drugs, and other practices that could be harmful to your health?

7. Do you participate in a regular exercise program or recreational activities?

8. Do you sleep well at night and wake up feeling refreshed and energized for the new day?

9. Are you actively involved in the religious organization of your choice, and do you take part in its youth activities?

10. Do you spend quality time with your family and friends in social and recreational activities?

11. Do you support family activities and efforts to maintain a good home life?

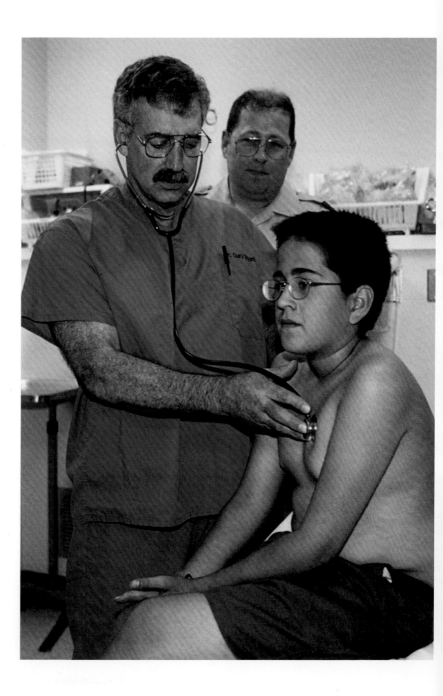

Maintaining Good Health

The first step in starting any personal fitness program is to get a physical examination from your doctor. Your dental health also affects your physical health, so a checkup from your dentist is also important. And to maintain your good health, you need to learn how to avoid diseases and other illness.

The Physical Exam

Before you fulfill the requirements for the Personal Fitness merit badge, have your health-care provider give you a physical exam. Be sure to use the BSA's Personal Health and Medical Record form. Use the form provided by your counselor or request the form from your local council service center. Your family physician probably has most of your personal information and medical history on file.

When you meet with your doctor, you will fill out a personal and medical questionnaire. It will ask about any diseases that are common in your family, your personal medical history, any allergic reactions to medicine, whether you are taking any medicine, and some personal information.

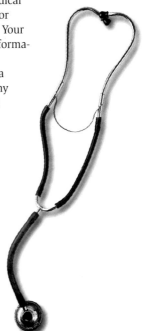

The physical examination will probably include

- Measuring your heart rate, blood pressure, height, and weight

- Checking heart and lung sounds

- Examining your ears, mouth, and throat

- Conducting an eye exam

- Testing your reflexes

The health-care professional should also ask questions and record observations about your psychosocial (mental and social) traits, nutritional habits, physical activity, and family circumstances. The physician will keep a permanent record of your health history, growth patterns, immunizations, and other data.

During a physical exam, your health-care provider may identify symptoms or conditions that need treatment or correction. It is wise to have regular physical exams so that your physician can monitor and keep a record of your health. The records are useful later in life when it is necessary to review your medical history.

"Average" and "Normal" Growth Rates

Your body type and rate of growth and development will be unique to you. In an average high school freshman class, for example, the height of the boys can range from 4 feet 8 inches to 6 feet tall. While the average height might be about 5 feet 4 inches, you probably will not find many "average" students who are precisely 5 feet 4 inches. Obviously, what is "normal" involves a wider range.

There is no reason for concern if you check charts and graphs and find results that do not match your measurements. These charts do not take into account your own special heredity and growth pattern. These are the main factors affecting growth, and they are never the same for any two people. Find out from your health-care provider what your position on the chart means.

Real growth problems are rare. Because of uncommon abnormalities, some people may grow excessively tall or fat. A person might be extraordinarily slow to mature or do so at an early age. If you regularly consult your doctor, there is probably no need to become concerned about growth problems. Your doctor will gladly answer any questions you have about your growth and maturity.

The Dental Exam and Daily Care of Your Teeth

For requirement 1b, you need to have a dental exam and get a statement from your dentist stating that your teeth have been checked and cared for. You also need to be able to tell your counselor how you properly care for your teeth on a daily basis.

Your dentist can tell if you have cavities or plaque buildup on your teeth and if your gums look healthy. Poor dental care can harm your health and your appearance. Proper daily care and regular dental checkups can help keep your teeth in good condition.

Although there is probably no single reason why teeth decay, you can do a few things to help protect your teeth. For example, a nutritious diet helps keep teeth in good condition. Usually, a diet that is good for general health is good for dental health. Do not fill up on pastries and sweets after or between meals. Sugary foods stick to teeth and cause them to decay over time.

Also, make it a habit to brush your teeth immediately after eating. If you cannot brush, rinse your mouth to get rid of food particles. When particles remain in your mouth, they form acids that attack your teeth and eventually form cavities. Toothpaste is helpful in cleaning, but thorough, proper brushing of all surfaces is the most important thing in preventing plaque buildup and fighting gum disease.

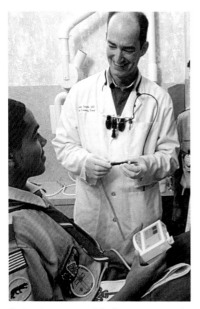

A dentist can explain how to properly care for your teeth.

Visit your dentist every six months and follow his or her advice. Keeping your teeth clean and avoiding gum disease can ensure an attractive smile and greatly enhance your general health.

How to Brush

Brush your teeth away from the gums instead of toward them. The brush should have a small head with firm but not hard bristles and a flat brushing surface. Most dentists also recommend flossing at least once a day. Flossing removes food particles and plaque between teeth and in the gums.

If the water you drink contains fluoride, your teeth will be more resistant to cavities. If it does not, ask your dentist whether you should use a dietary supplement. You can also use a toothpaste that contains fluoride. Studies have shown that using toothpaste with fluoride helps prevent tooth decay.

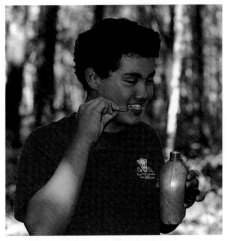

Scouts can still care for their teeth at a campsite.

Your dentist may also discuss your *occlusion,* or bite. If your teeth do not close on each other properly, they may wear down quickly and you may develop other dental troubles. Your dentist will tell you if your teeth need to be straightened.

Because of recent advances in dental care, gum disease now causes more tooth loss than actual tooth decay. It is also now believed that bacteria that cause gum disease can harm the tissue and muscles of the heart, so flossing and other measures to help prevent gum disease may also protect your cardiovascular health. Talk to your dental professional about how to prevent gum disease.

Disease Prevention

Your body is an amazingly complex creation. Learn to listen to your body so that you can recognize its warning signs. Most illnesses have recognizable symptoms. When your body shows symptoms, it generally means something is wrong. Heed the warning signs. Consult your health-care provider when symptoms appear. Your doctor depends on your accurate description of what you are feeling to diagnose the disease or illness so that proper treatment can be given.

Some diseases are entirely preventable, so regular visits to your health-care provider are important. He or she can advise you in preventive habits. Your daily habits may expose you to people with a contagious disease or make you more susceptible to certain diseases.

Poor eating habits weaken your body and make you susceptible to colds and flu. Muscles and bones weak from inactivity may make you more vulnerable to injuries. Not dressing warmly in wet and cold weather may increase your chances of catching a cold or the flu.

A Scout Is Clean

Keeping your body clean by showering daily and washing your hands with soap and warm water several times a day can help prevent you from picking up or spreading airborne diseases such as flu and colds. It is also important to wash your hands after each and every time you go to the bathroom.

Never drink from someone else's cup. Cover your mouth when you sneeze or cough, and use tissues. Always use clean drinking and eating utensils. Being around people who are sick may expose you to communicable viruses or bacteria. If someone is sick, keep your distance.

Primary prevention involves developing good health habits and changing bad ones, or preventing bad habits from forming. This means taking measures to combat risk factors for illness before an illness actually develops. (See "Risk Factors" later in this chapter.)

Primary prevention is a good idea, but it is not always easy to put into practice. For one thing, people often have little immediate reason to watch out for their health. So they allow themselves to form bad habits that may be hard to overcome. When health habits develop in a person's youth, most people are healthy. The damage that bad habits like smoking, drinking alcohol, and using drugs cause to all organs of the body may not show up for many years.

When you are young, it is sometimes difficult to understand that the habits you develop now may influence whether you develop major health problems later on. Think of your body as a well-running car engine: With proper care and maintenance, that car will run smoothly for a long time. With your body, you want it to run smoothly and be problem-free for many decades. So now is the time to start taking good care of yourself and making sure your body, mind, and spirit get what is needed to not just survive—but to thrive.

Unfortunately, even good habits and youth cannot prevent all diseases. A person with a healthy lifestyle can still be struck with a serious disease or die unexpectedly. Symptoms may not always be obvious, making the disease hard to detect. In other cases, symptoms are simply ignored. But now is the best time for you to develop good habits for your overall health.

Immunizations

Having immunization shots during childhood minimizes your risk of getting many dangerous diseases, such as the following.

- **Diphtheria,** an infectious disease affecting the membranes of the nose and throat, results in fever, pain, and respiratory obstructions. The toxins (poisons) that cause diphtheria may also cause myocarditis (inflammation of the heart).

- **Pertussis** is the medical name for whooping cough, an infectious disease that causes severe and rapid coughing.

- **Tetanus** is an often-fatal disease marked by general muscular spasms and vocal cord spasms, seizures, respiratory spasms, and paralysis. The toxin that causes the disease enters the body through wounds. For example, if you step on a rusty nail and drive it into your foot, you could get tetanus if you do not get immunized for this disease.

- **Meningitis** is an inflammation of the membranes surrounding the brain and spinal cord.

- **Polio** is a viral disease that may result in muscle atrophy, paralysis, and/or permanent deformity.

The ages at which children and young adults should receive vaccines and boosters are shown in the table. Because of the risk of being infected with the tetanus toxin through open wounds, the tetanus shot is given every 10 years, even through adulthood.

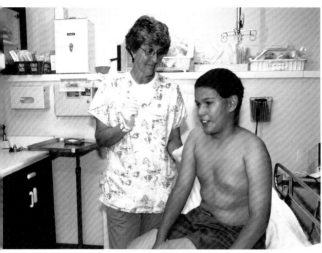

Immunization shots are important for the prevention of some diseases.

Recommended Immunizations for Children in the United States*

Age	Vaccine
Birth	Hepatitis B (first dose)
1 to 4 months	Hepatitis B (second dose)
6 to 18 months	Hepatitis B (third dose); inactivated poliovirus
12 to 15 months	*Haemophilus influenzae* type b; mumps, measles, rubella (first dose); pneumococcal
12 to 18 months	Varicella
12 months through 18 years	Influenza (annually)
15 to 18 months	Diptheria, tetanus, and pertussis
24 months to 18 years	Hepatitis A series

*Source: Centers for Disease Control and Prevention, Advisory Committee on Immunization Practices

Other Preventable Diseases

The disease *acquired immunodeficiency syndrome (AIDS)* is generating great concern worldwide. AIDS damages the immune system of the body. This damage prevents the immune system from fighting infections, diseases caused by bacteria or viruses, and life-threatening diseases such as cancer, meningitis, and pneumonia. The disease is most often spread by sexual contact and intravenous drug needles and syringes. However, it also can be transmitted through blood transfusions.

Because the immune system is out of order, people with AIDS can die from diseases that normally could be treated. Unfortunately, AIDS patients often do not respond to treatment. The medical community has made progress in discovering drugs to treat AIDS, but no drug has yet been fully proven or accepted as safe or successful. To date, there is no real cure for AIDS—only prevention, which emphasizes measures such as staying away from drugs and avoiding sexual contact without personal protection measures.

Rheumatic fever is another disease that can be prevented with better understanding of good health practices. Rheumatic fever starts with a simple throat infection that leads to strep throat. Left untreated, the disease may affect the joints and even the heart. Symptoms include sore throat, fever, fatigue, and pale complexion.

Not many people with strep throat get rheumatic fever, but if a sore throat lasts for several days, consult your doctor. A simple throat culture can diagnose strep throat and rheumatic fever can be prevented. Rheumatic fever that progresses to the point of heart damage becomes a permanent disease.

Risk Factors

The medical community does not know what causes many diseases. But in the case of cancer and heart disease, years of research and observation have revealed behaviors that increase the risk of getting the diseases. These behaviors are called *risk factors.*

Risk factors such as age, gender, or race cannot be changed. Other risk factors such as dietary habits, too much sun exposure, lack of physical activity, excessive mental stress, and smoking can be modified.

Risk factors for heart disease that may exist during adolescence include:

- Obesity
- Sex (males are at higher risk)
- High blood pressure
- High blood cholesterol
- Diabetes
- Smoking
- Lack of exercise
- Family history of heart disease

The greatest cause of death and disabilities in the United States is coronary (heart) disease. It is responsible for about 500,000 deaths each year. On average, three Americans suffer a heart attack every minute. Many people can reduce this risk through lifestyle changes.

Exercise alone will not prevent or cure heart disease, but it is one effective way to reduce the risk of cardiovascular (heart and blood vessel) disease. Inactive people have twice the risk of heart attack compared with those who regularly exercise. But only exercises that significantly increase the blood flow to the working muscles for extended periods promote cardiovascular fitness.

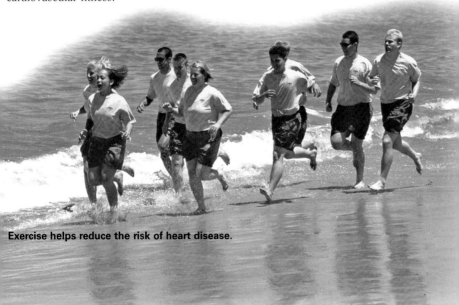

Exercise helps reduce the risk of heart disease.

This type of exercise is called "aerobic," which means the body uses oxygen to produce the energy that is needed for the activity. Running, swimming, and biking are good examples of aerobic exercises that get your heart rate up and increase blood flow to muscles. Strengthening exercises, such as weight and resistance training, help build muscles and tone your body but do little to promote cardiovascular fitness.

Obesity in children and teenagers has now reached epidemic proportions. Obesity in young people is caused, in part, by the many hours they spend each day in front of the television or computer, added to eating far too many high-fat, high-calorie foods and fast food.

Obesity greatly increases the likelihood of developing low self-esteem, depression, high blood pressure, high cholesterol levels, and diabetes—major risk factors. Childhood obesity leads to adult obesity. The risk of death from cardiovascular disease is much higher for people who were obese in childhood. Therefore, treatment of childhood and adolescent obesity—through exercise and proper diet—is incredibly important in preventing severe disease in adulthood.

Although hanging out on the couch and eating foods that are bad for you represents a significant risk factor, smoking triples your risk of developing cardiovascular disease. The good

Try cycling with friends instead of hanging out on the couch and watching TV. Your heart will thank you.

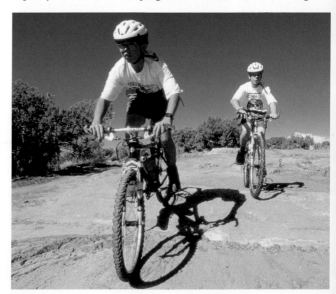

news is that recent studies have shown the body has an amazing ability to repair itself once a person stops smoking. Within two weeks of stopping, your body will respond by becoming healthier. Within a few years, your lung capacity (that is, your ability to breathe easy) will nearly double.

Cancer—Seven Danger Signs

If you recognize any of these seven danger signs, seek further testing for cancer. Awareness of these seven signs will increase the chances of diagnosing cancer at an early stage and therefore increase your chance of survival.

1. Change in bowel or bladder habits could be a sign of colorectal cancer.

2. A sore that does not heal on the skin or in the mouth could be a malignancy and should be checked by a doctor.

3. Unusual bleeding or discharge from the rectum or bladder could mean colorectal, prostate, or bladder cancer.

4. Thickening of breast tissue or a new lump in the breast is a warning sign of breast cancer. A lump in the testes could mean testicular cancer.

5. Indigestion or trouble swallowing could be cancer of the mouth, throat, esophagus, or stomach.

6. Obvious changes to moles or warts could mean skin cancer.

7. Nagging cough or hoarseness that persists for four to six weeks could be a sign of lung or throat cancer.

Closely watch for these signs, which are your body's way of alerting you to potential problems. If you experience any of them, schedule an appointment with your physician immediately.

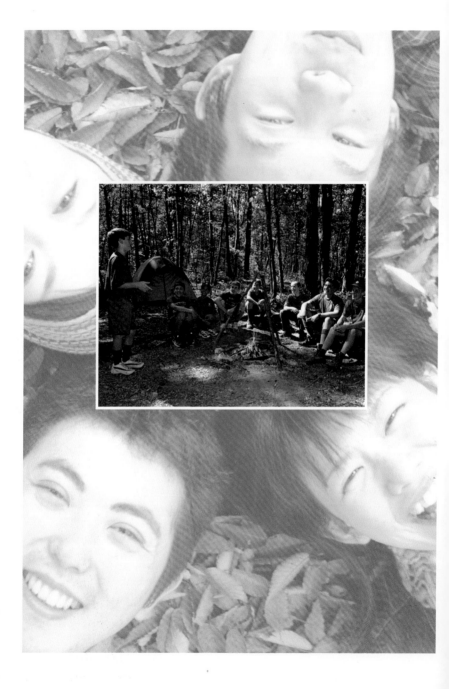

Social, Emotional, Mental, and Spiritual Fitness

Living the Scout Oath and Law, the Scout motto, and the Scout slogan helps every Scout live a healthy life. What would your social interaction be if you were not trustworthy, loyal, helpful, friendly, courteous, kind, obedient, cheerful, thrifty, brave, clean, and reverent? In obeying the Scout Law, you should try to show those personal qualities every day, in all situations, and with everyone you meet. By taking the Scout Oath, you promise to obey the Scout Law and to help others at all times. The Scout who is recognized as a Scout by his actions rather than by a uniform has truly lived the Scout Law.

You know now that living the Scout Law affects your social fitness. To understand why, think what each point of the Scout Law means. Review the Scout Oath and Scout Law in your *Boy Scout Handbook* or at the back of this pamphlet.

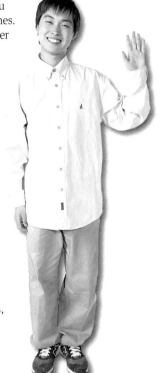

Social Skills

There are many things to consider in developing good social skills. Making friends is easy if you extend yourself in an open and engaging way. Remember that everyone is different but almost everyone has interesting and unique qualities.

Think about the characteristics you value in a good friend. Your friends value some of the same characteristics in you. Good friends share feelings and emotions with trust and confidence. Everyone needs someone to talk to about his or her feelings, emotions, and problems, as well as someone to have fun with. Friends help one another through bad and good times and are able to speak honestly to one another.

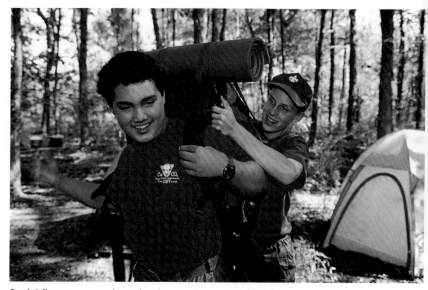

Social fitness means knowing how to be a good friend.

Good communication requires two people—a talker and a listener. These are not skills that come naturally; they need to be learned. When you express your feelings and emotions, it is important to express them appropriately. When you listen, do so with sincerity and concern for your friend's feelings and problems. By sharing your own feelings and emotions, you allow others to become involved with your life. And by being a good listener, you can help others to confront problems, emotions, and struggles in their lives.

Being a good listener is just part of being a good friend. Accepting others is important to your social health as well as to theirs. Everyone, including you, has the need to be accepted. You do not need to approve of a person's behavior, but you can accept him or her as an individual. Friends do not judge each other but accept each other unconditionally.

Peer Pressure

Dealing with peer pressure is tough. You will not always be fortunate enough to have acquaintances who are positive influences in your life and share the same values and standards that you have. You can accept these people as individuals without doing what they do. You cannot stop peer pressure, but do not allow

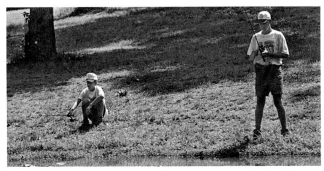

It is important for good friends to spend time with each other; it helps strengthen friendships by building understanding, trust, and respect.

people to tease you or push you to join activities that make you uncomfortable or that are unlawful.

For example, your friends might try to get you to go swimming in a dangerous rock quarry where swimming is not allowed. You could do one of two things. You could walk away from the situation or offer another activity that is more appropriate, such as going to the public swimming pool. By walking away, you show your unwillingness to participate, but by offering an alternative, you are providing positive leadership. If your friends do not accept your alternative, you can still walk away. If they accept your suggestion, chances are that everyone will have just as much fun at the pool and will be much safer.

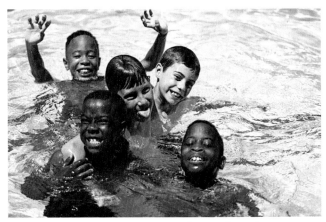

Always swim with a friend where a lifeguard is on duty.

Know Your Priorities

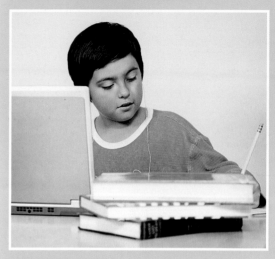

For your own social well-being, it is helpful to list your priorities. Your priorities will be different from someone else's. Your list might include yourself, your family, religion, friends, education, recreation, health, and work. *You* should be the first priority. You cannot help others, do Good Turns daily, or be a friend if you neglect your own body, mind, and spiritual needs.

Always try to help others raise their own standards and do the right thing. Do not stand back and watch your friends make the wrong decisions. You may feel as if you are all alone at times when facing peer pressure. But rest assured that staying true to your values as a Scout will make a long-lasting impression on others.

Some young people suffer from low self-esteem, low self-confidence, and insecurity. Some kids are too strict with themselves, expecting perfection. They may try to be like someone else because that person seems to attract friends. This may lead to behavior that removes them from achieving their potential.

You do not need to choose drugs, smoking, or harmful behavior. If you know you are taking good care of your body, accepting responsibility, taking pride in your accomplishments, living the Scout Oath and Law, and participating in healthy activities with friends and family, then you probably feel good about yourself and what you are doing. Although peer acceptance is important, your self-esteem, self-confidence, and sense of identity ultimately come from within.

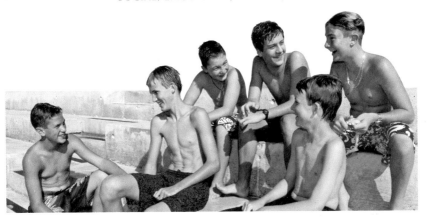

Emotional Fitness

Your emotional well-being is closely tied to the other components of personal fitness. Your activities, exercise, diet, sleep, family life, religious involvement, and physical health all affect your emotional and mental fitness. Everyone worries a little. It is normal to have some temporary anxiety or depression while overcoming major transitions or obstacles in life. But if anxiety and worry are excessive and interfere with school, family, friendships, and a healthy social life, you should seek professional help.

Positive activities with friends help maintain good emotional fitness.

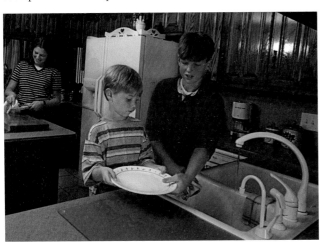

Helping with chores is an important contribution to a happy family life.

Many emotional problems can be prevented in the home. A good family life is essential to a healthy mind and body. Not every family is the same. Some Scouts have parents who are divorced or deceased. These boys can have a happy home life with a single parent or guardian. As a family member, your contributions are important to your family's well-being. Support family efforts for a peaceful and meaningful home life. Just as your parents help you overcome your problems, you can help overcome some family problems.

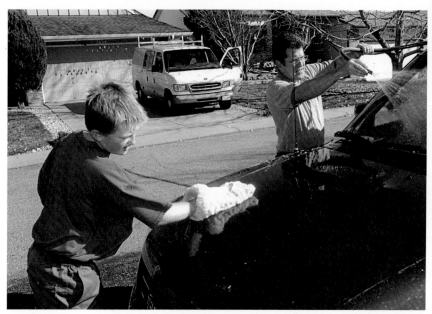

Be a friend to your family. Your contributions are important to your family's well-being.

Help plan family outings and activities. Spend quality time with your brothers, sisters, and parents. "Quality time" means sharing through communication and joint activity. If you talk about common interests, work together on a family project, plan for a special occasion, share a pleasant or meaningful experience, or play together, you are getting and giving healthy benefits through your family activity. Your family can be your most important possession.

Earlier you learned that being a good communicator means being able to express your emotions and feelings to a good friend. This friend might be your parent, your Scoutmaster, a brother or sister, another Scout, or your religious leader.

Of course, you must be aware of your feelings and emotions to be able to express them. Examining your feelings is the first step. For example, if you have ever been in a situation like the one at the rock quarry described previously, how did you feel? Be honest. Were you disappointed in your friends? Ashamed? Angry? Your feelings are your own and should be expressed as such. When you talk to your friend, say, "I felt angry when they asked me to go with them. They know we should not go there." Do not say, "They made me angry." It is healthy to admit your feelings, but remember that they are *your* feelings. No one made you feel that way.

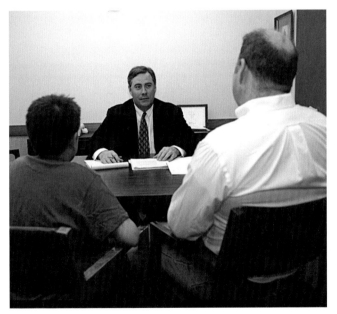

Professional counselors can help people facing difficult emotional issues.

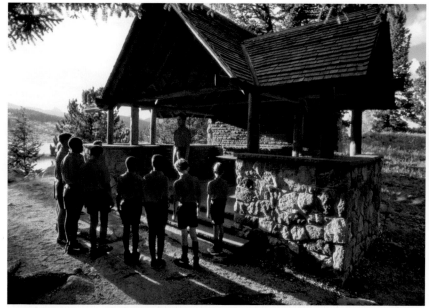

Your religious practices will help you to live by the Scout Law.

Spiritual Fitness

The Boy Scouts of America is an integral part of nearly every place of worship. This is because every Scout has a duty to God. A troop that is chartered to a religious group provides Scouts the opportunity to recognize and fulfill their duty. Active involvement in your religious group is essential to your being a good Scout. You are expected to recognize your duty to God, and the religious principles you learn will enable you to live by the Scout Law.

Religions around the world use Scouting as a way to provide meaningful activities for young men. Most of them have special recognitions for the young people who recognize and fulfill their duty to God. Some of these emblems are the Ad Altare Dei, Alpha Omega, God and Country, Living Faith, Ner Tamid, and On My Honor. Check with your religious leaders to find out the requirements for receiving the emblem affiliated with your religion. Religious emblems are not required for advancement but are honorable to wear on your uniform and demonstrate your dedication to your religion and to Scouting.

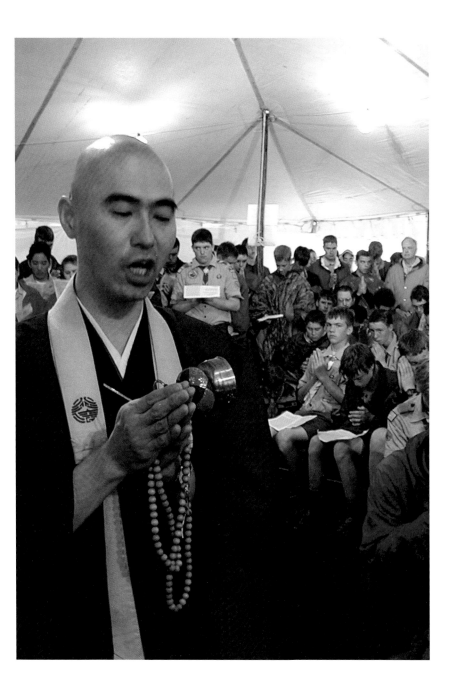

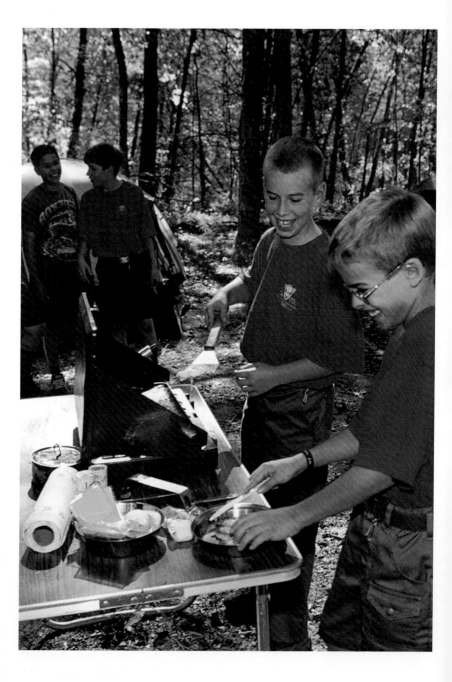

Eating Right: Good Nutrition Made Easy

Eating right plays an important role in all components of personal fitness. If your body does not get the nutrients it needs, it will not function at its best. Eating foods that are bad for you may result in lack of energy, slow healing of injuries, dehydration, excessive weight loss, or buildup of body fat.

The word "diet" does not always mean cutting back on calories to lose weight. Your diet is what you eat every day, whether you are trying to lose, maintain, or gain weight.

Many illnesses are affected by diet. Failure to eat properly may be fatal for a person with diabetes. Good nutrition is especially important for people at risk for, or diagnosed with, heart disease. Many people with mild high blood pressure can lower it by eating less salt and fewer calories. People can often lower their blood cholesterol levels by increasing exercise and reducing the amount of fat, cholesterol, and calories they consume.

Diet is also important for people with cancer. Many scientists believe that foods such as broccoli, cabbage, carrots, cauliflower, fruits, spinach, whole-grain breads and cereals, and some seafoods contain substances that may help prevent some cancers. Eating less fat and more fiber may also help prevent some cancers.

> Variety is not only the spice of life, it is important to your overall health. A balanced diet includes all the food groups.

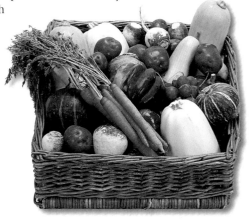

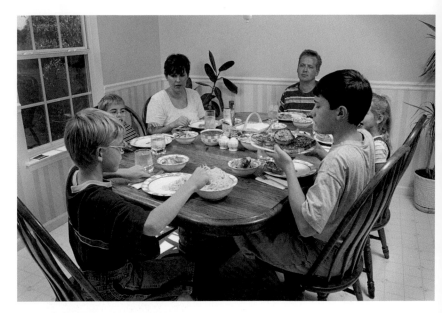

Nutrients

The key to good nutrition is to eat a varied diet.

A healthy diet provides six basic nutrients: protein, fat, carbohydrates, water, vitamins, and minerals. Eating a variety of foods will provide your body with all the nutrients needed for good health.

Protein is essential to every cell in the body for growth and repair of damaged tissue. The body needs protein to make the antibodies (disease fighters) that increase your resistance to disease. Protein is not stored in the body like other nutrients, so it is important to eat protein-rich foods each day. But your body can use only small amounts of protein at one time.

Fat is also an important nutrient. It is part of cell walls. Fatty deposits support and cushion vital organs in your body. Fat also acts as an insulator. Even so, too much fat in your diet can cause obesity. Dietary fat comes from cooking oils, butter, margarine, salad oils, meat, nuts, eggs, chocolate, olives, fried foods, mayonnaise, avocados, and gravies. Good sources of healthy unsaturated fat include olive oil, canola, soy, corn, sunflower, peanut, and other vegetable oils, as well as fatty fish such as salmon.

Carbohydrates (sugars and starches) are the main source of energy for your muscles and nervous system, especially during exercise. Simple carbohydrates—sugars—add flavor to foods and yield high energy in the body. Foods high in sugar often have many calories but few nutrients. Nutritionists sometimes call them "empty calorie" foods. Avoid these types of foods, or eat them only in moderation. Complex carbohydrates, such as whole-grain products, are digested more slowly, provide energy over a longer time, and are less harmful to your teeth.

Water is essential to life. Your body is about 60 percent water. Water helps to regulate body temperature and aids in digestion. Water is also important in just about every chemical reaction in your body. Daily water losses need to be replaced continually. Eight glasses of water a day is recommended.

Vitamins are the most frequently talked about nutrient because most people believe they are important and good for them. Unfortunately, people also have the notion that "if a little is good, then more is better." Taking a daily multivitamin supplement will help ensure that your body gets all the nutrients it needs.

Minerals such as calcium, iron, iodine, potassium, and magnesium have specific purposes in the body. Minerals are excreted after they are used. For a balanced diet, minerals must be continually replaced through proper diet and daily supplements.

Drink water with meals and snacks rather than drinking soda pop.

Physically strong choon

Food Groups

Foods are classified into basic food groups: grains, fruits, vegetables, meats and beans, dairy foods, and fats and sweets. Foods in the same category provide similar nutrients.

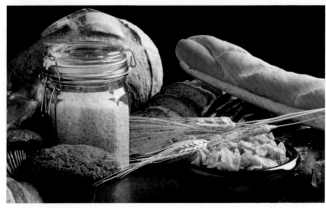

Foods made from whole grains are healthier than foods made from refined grains.

Whole grains such as whole-wheat bread, brown rice, oatmeal, and whole-grain pastas and cereals are the major dietary sources of carbohydrates. Grains contribute significant amounts of minerals, vitamins, and carbohydrates. These nutrients keep blood sugar and insulin levels from rising, then falling, too quickly. By better controlling blood sugar and insulin, you can keep hunger at bay. These foods may prevent the development of type 2 diabetes.

You should have vegetables and fruits two to three times a day, or at nearly every meal.

The **vegetable and fruit groups** include fresh, frozen, canned, and dried forms. These foods provide many of the essential vitamins. Vitamins A and C are commonly found in vegetables and fruits. These great-tasting foods protect against a variety of cancers, lower blood pressure, and can decrease your chances of having heart problems.

The **fish, poultry, and eggs group** is the most important provider of protein. Eating fish periodically can reduce your chances of heart disease. Chicken and turkey are also good sources of protein and can be low in saturated fat. Eggs, which are also a good source of protein, contain higher levels of cholesterol. But eggs are still better than eating a doughnut or a bagel made from refined flour for breakfast.

The **red meat and butter group** foods contain a lot of saturated fat. Foods in this group should be eaten sparingly. If you eat red meat every day, switching to fish and chicken several times a week can lower your cholesterol levels. Switching from butter to olive oil can do the same thing.

The **nuts and beans group** is another source of protein. This group also provides fiber, vitamins, and minerals. Legumes include black beans, navy beans, garbanzos, and other types of beans. Many kinds of nuts such as almonds, walnuts, pecans, peanuts, hazelnuts, and pistachios contain healthy fats.

The **dairy group** includes low-fat milk, cheese, low-fat cottage cheese, yogurt, puddings, creamed soups, and ice cream. Dairy products provide calcium for the body and are often fortified with vitamins A and D. While dairy products also provide fat in your diet, skim milk and low-fat cheese provide healthy alter-natives. If you enjoy dairy foods, which provide bone-building calcium, and you need vitamin D, stick with no-fat or low-fat products. Calcium supplements are another way to get your daily calcium if your body cannot handle milk products.

Remember: Eat fats and sweets sparingly because they often provide little or no nutritional value and are high in calories.

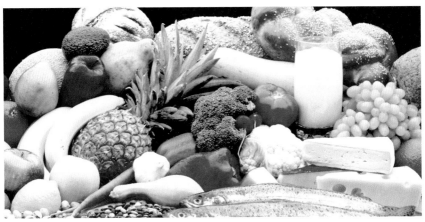

A balanced diet includes all the food groups.

Foods in the **white rice, white bread, potatoes, pasta, and sweets category** should also be eaten sparingly. They cause fast increases in blood sugar that can lead to weight gain, diabetes, heart disease, and other health disorders. Whole-grain carbohydrates cause slower, steadier increases in blood sugar that do not overwhelm your body.

The Food Pyramid

The federal government's food pyramid helps people better understand what they should eat and how much they should consume each day to be healthy.

A rainbow of colored, vertical stripes in the pyramid represents the five food groups, as well as fats and oils. The colors stand for the following food groups:

❶ **Orange**—grains

❷ **Green**—vegetables

❸ **Red**—fruits

❹ **Yellow**—fats and oils

❺ **Blue**—milk and dairy products

❻ **Purple**—meat, beans, fish, and nuts

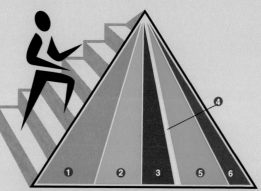

MyPyramid.gov
STEPS TO A HEALTHIER YOU

Notice the person climbing the stairway up the side of the pyramid. That is to show how important it is to be active and exercise. You can make changes one step at a time to be healthier. The content of the pyramid changes depending on whether you are a girl or boy, what age you are, and how much exercise you get on a daily basis. With your parent's permission, go to *http://www.mypyramid.gov* to figure out what your pyramid looks like.

Eat less of some foods and more of others. The bands in the pyramid for meat and protein (purple) and oils (yellow) are thinner than the other bands because you need less of those foods than you do fruits, vegetables, grains, and dairy foods.

Energy and Calories

The foods you eat provide energy for your body when they are broken down in your stomach or intestinal tract, absorbed into the bloodstream, and stored in the cells of your body. When your body demands energy, stored supplies of carbohydrates or fats are broken down and transported to the cells that require energy. In the cells, carbohydrates (in the form of sugar) and fats are used in chemical processes that release energy. The energy released causes muscles to contract. Energy also is used to carry on other bodily functions, including those of your stomach and digestive tract, liver, kidneys, and nervous system. Your heart beats all the time, even while you sleep, and needs a constant supply of energy.

Your body's energy needs are spoken of as *calories*. Only carbohydrates, fats, and proteins provide calories in your diet. Although foods contain vitamins and minerals, these elements do not provide calories. Water also has no calories. Labels tell how many grams of carbohydrates, fat, and protein are in food. Labels also list total calories.

Carbohydrates have 4 calories per gram, fats have 9 calories per gram, and proteins have 4 calories per gram. It would almost seem logical that it would be better to eat more fatty foods since they provide the most energy (calories). Gram for gram, they do provide the most energy, but eating lots of fat can cause many problems. Excess dietary fat can lead to various cardiovascular diseases as well as obesity.

The quality of calories is just as important as the proper quantity of calories. Receiving 1,000 calories from empty-calorie foods and 1,000 calories from a well-balanced diet is not the same. Both plans provide 1,000 calories, but only the balanced diet will provide the required vitamins and minerals.

The more intense an exercise, the more calories you need. If you were to walk and run for the same amount of time, running would require the most calories. How long the exercise lasts (its duration) also has an impact on caloric requirements. If you were to exercise for 20 minutes one day and then do the same type of exercise the next day for 30 minutes, you would need more calories to carry out the exercise for 30 minutes.

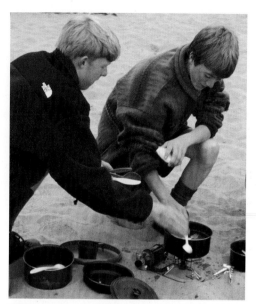

With planning, healthy meals can be prepared even in the wilderness.

To monitor your food intake, it is necessary to be aware of your body. If you are not eating enough, you may feel lazy and tired. You will not have enough energy to participate in many activities. You also may be more vulnerable to colds and flu.

If you are constantly eating more than your energy needs, you may feel bloated and uncomfortable. Over time, you may notice a weight gain. Weight gain is often slow enough that you do not notice it right away. In fact, you may not notice until you put on a favorite shirt and discover your clothing does not fit anymore.

Weight control is more than just maintaining an ideal body weight throughout your life. Weight control involves fat control. If you are inactive and eat poorly, your body composition may have a large portion of fat. If you are active, exercise regularly, and eat nutritious meals, though your body weight may be the same as that of someone who is fatter, your body composition may be ideal for you.

Some people (athletes, for example) may weigh more but are lean. Other people might not weigh as much but can still be classified as obese. With respect to how you look and feel, it is better to think in terms of "fat control" rather than "weight control."

Behavior Modification

Exercise and good nutrition are two of the elements of weight control; the other is *behavior modification.* When used together, these three components can help you control the amount of fat on your body. By eating properly, your dietary intake will be balanced and adequate in calories. By exercising, you will use the calories that you consume and shrink your percentage of body fat. Exercising also builds stronger muscles and greater muscular endurance, and it increases cardiovascular endurance.

Most vegetables, grains, and fruits are high in nutrition and low in fat compared with dairy products and meats. Emphasize the high-priority foods when planning meals and snacks. Remember that it is important to eat a well-balanced diet of foods from all food groups. Serve yourself smaller portions to begin your meal. Eat until you are comfortably full, then stop.

Good Snacks Help Build Better Bodies

For some people, snacking between meals is a good idea. In fact, it is healthier to eat a light snack between breakfast and lunch, and between lunch and dinner. Of course, nutritious snacks are best, and too much snacking will spoil your appetite for a healthy lunch or dinner. Snack on fruit or finger vegetables such as celery and carrots. Try not to eat just because you are bored. You could easily devour a whole bag of potato chips or half a bag of cookies when you are watching television or doing homework. Make a point to notice what you are eating and how much.

Exercise at least 30 minutes a day to reduce the risk of chronic disease. Increase your exercise program to 60 minutes daily to prevent weight gain and up to 90 minutes daily if you have lost weight and want to keep it off.

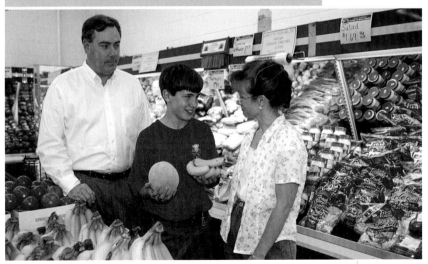

A menu plan not only helps you prepare nutritious meals, but also helps cut down on the expense of unplanned food purchases.

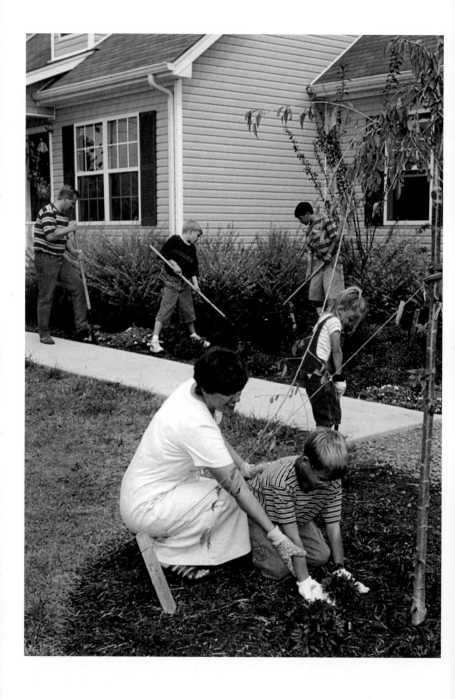

Physical Fitness

Physical fitness means different things to different people. In general, *physical fitness* is the ability to do vigorous physical work without undue fatigue. A physically fit person has energy left over to enjoy daily recreational and social activities and to meet the energy demands of unforeseen emergencies.

Physical fitness includes the following four components:

1. Cardiovascular and pulmonary endurance

2. Muscular strength and endurance

3. Flexibility

4. Body composition

A personal physical fitness program is important because the ordinary tasks of daily living do not provide enough regular vigorous exercise to maintain good body composition, cardiovascular endurance, or muscle tone.

Several studies have shown that young people and adults in the United States lack physical fitness. Most adults do not exercise regularly, and school-age children (ages 6 through 17) have become less fit in recent years. Today's young people generally have more body fat and perform worse in cardiovascular endurance events than youth in the past.

The President's Council on Physical Fitness and Health reports that children and teens today have poorer physical fitness than those of 20 years ago. Many young people cannot run a mile or do even a single push-up. These things are important because having physical problems in your childhood often carry over into adulthood. As a young person, you develop the habits and attitudes that you will carry with you as an adult. Choose now the kind of lifestyle you want to have.

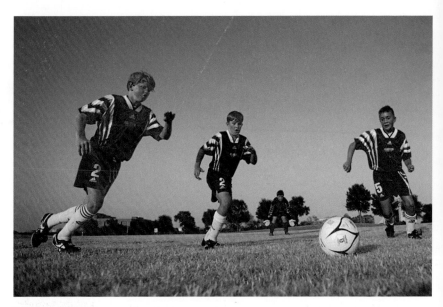

Team sports are a great way to combine exercise and fun.

No matter how physically fit you are now, you need to know why, how, and when to start an exercise program. The benefits of exercise include weight control, less stress, better muscular tone, greater cardiovascular endurance, greater flexibility, a better self-image, and just feeling good about yourself and about the way you look.

Mapping Out a Course

Ask your parent or guardian to help you map out a 1-mile course around your neighborhood by driving you in a vehicle so you can check the odometer reading. Once you and your parent have selected a safe course, go out and walk or run that mile.

Create an index card for each week and write how long it takes you to complete that mile every day you walk or run the course. Keep your record posted on your refrigerator so you can see your progress. You and your parents will be amazed at the results.

If you have to walk most of the course the first few days, do not be discouraged. Just try to run a little more of your route each day. You will be amazed at how quickly you can progress from barely being able to walk and run a mile to breezing through it and adding more miles to your daily routine.

Your lung capacity will expand, your energy level will soar, and you will find yourself creating a good habit that you will want to stick with because you will be able to *see* and *feel* the results. To get rid of a bad habit, replace it with a good habit. For instance, if you have a bad habit, such as eating too much, replace the time you would spend doing that with running. You will be much more successful if you trade a bad habit for a good one. Persevere! You are worth it.

Handling a Side Stitch

If you experience a condition called "side stitch" when running, do not be alarmed. Slow down to a slow jog, then breathe deeply in through your nose and out through your mouth until the side stitch goes away. Normally, you can run through this minor discomfort as long as you breathe deeply and correctly when you run.

Cardiovascular Endurance

Cardiovascular endurance is the ability to maintain an activity that is aerobic in nature. *Aerobic exercises* are defined as those exercises that involve a large portion of your body's muscle mass and are continuous and rhythmic. Aerobic exercises are used mainly for fun and to reduce stress, control weight, and improve cardiovascular endurance. Your body adapts to regular aerobic exercise in about six to eight weeks. Adaptations that help reduce stress happen quickly. Adaptations that help reduce fat and control weight take a little longer.

To decrease the chances of cramping, delay your exercise for an hour or two after a meal.

No single aerobic exercise is best suited for everyone. The best exercise for you is the one that you enjoy, and that you have opportunity to do, including access to any necessary facilities or equipment.

Exercises differ in the muscle groups they use. While running, walking, and bicycling use mainly leg muscles, swimming also uses back and arm muscles. Many health professionals consider swimming to be a superior aerobic exercise because it is a full-body, no-impact activity.

When choosing an exercise, you must first consider your purpose in exercising. Then choose an appropriate exercise that is fun and that you can do regularly. Cross-training—varying your workouts to strengthen both the muscular and the cardiovascular systems—helps prevent injury and boredom or burnout from too much repetition.

Aerobic Exercises Get You Moving

Types of aerobic exercises include walking, backpacking, bicycling, aerobic dance, jogging, running, and swimming. Different types of aerobic exercises vary greatly in intensity, or the difficulty of the exercise.

An exercise
program is
progressive.
Start out slowly.

After you choose an exercise, determine how much to exercise. Follow these guidelines for improving or maintaining cardiovascular fitness:

- Exercise regularly using aerobic activities.
- Exercise at least three to five times each week.
- Exercise 30 to 60 minutes each time.
- Exercise at an intensity that is 60 to 85 percent of your maximum heart rate.

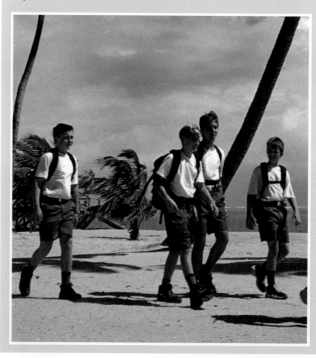

It is important to exercise correctly. Remember that an exercise program is progressive. Let's use running as an example. You might not be able to run for 20 minutes continuously the first day. If you need to, start out the first few days just walking. Then alternate several minutes of running and walking. In a few weeks, you will be running the entire 20 minutes. Remember, start slowly! Do not forget to warm up and stretch.

The intensity of the exercise is *inversely related* to the amount of time you can continue the exercise. In other words, if you jog slowly, you may be able to exercise for 20 minutes at first. But if you were to sprint, you might last only a few minutes.

You should have a sense of how you feel when you are exercising. Do not exhaust yourself. Pace yourself to finish the 20 minutes. A good running pace is a "run-talk" pace, slow enough that you can carry on a conversation with someone running beside you. If you are running too fast, you will be too tired and unable to talk comfortably.

> The harder you exercise, the higher your heart rate, and the less time you will be able to continue the exercise.

Another way to monitor your intensity is to check your heart rate about five minutes after you start exercising. To do this, stop exercising and place the index and middle finger of your right hand on the radial artery of your left wrist. When you feel the heartbeat pulsations, count the number of beats you feel in 15 seconds. Multiply the number of beats you count by four to get your heartbeat per minute. Your exercising heart rate should be between 125 and 170 beats per minute.

The first few minutes of exercise may seem uncomfortable because it takes a few minutes for your body to adjust each time you exercise. You can lessen the initial discomfort by starting with an appropriate warm-up.

A suitable warm-up includes five to 10 minutes of low-intensity movements followed by several minutes of stretching exercises. If you run, your warm-up may include walking or a slow jog. Warm-up activities help decrease the chance of injury and increase blood flow to active muscles, body temperature, and metabolism (the chemical processes that release energy in the body). All these changes help make for a smoother flow into your exercise.

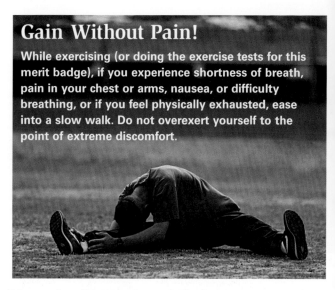

Gain Without Pain!

While exercising (or doing the exercise tests for this merit badge), if you experience shortness of breath, pain in your chest or arms, nausea, or difficulty breathing, or if you feel physically exhausted, ease into a slow walk. Do not overexert yourself to the point of extreme discomfort.

Include stretching exercises in your warm-up.

Muscular Strength and Endurance

Muscular strength is the ability of your muscles to contract and exert force against an opposing force. Muscular strength is usually measured in terms of how much force your muscles can exert—for example, lifting a certain amount of weight.

Muscular endurance is the ability of your muscles to contract repeatedly or hold a contraction against an opposing force. For example, hiking up a mountain or carrying supplies to a camp requires great muscular endurance. Every activity you do requires some muscular strength and endurance.

Strengthening exercises such as weight lifting build denser, stronger bones and will help a person maintain bone density later in life. These types of exercises can also enhance coordination and reaction time, and build stronger ligaments and joints to help prevent injury. Strong muscles also help support the bony structures of your body and help with good posture.

Maintaining strong muscles throughout your life will let you take part in more activities when you get older. Many people lower their physical activity so much as they age that muscles weaken quickly and stop them from doing simple household chores.

The abdominal muscles are some of the most neglected muscles of the body. Weak abdominal muscles are a major cause of lower back pain. This muscle weakness also may contribute to spinal curvature abnormalities, poor posture, and a bulging belly. Strong abdominal muscles help support the spine and maintain good posture.

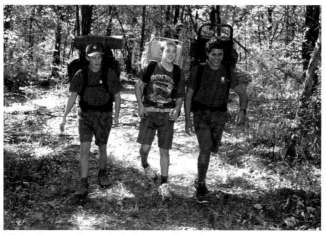

Hiking is a great way to build muscle endurance.

You do not need an expensive weight room or a health club to do strengthening exercises. Sit-ups, push-ups, and pull-ups are great exercises to strengthen your shoulders, chest, back, arms, and abdomen. Spending 10 to 20 minutes each day doing these three exercises will make a difference.

Start by seeing how many sit-ups, push-ups, and pull-ups you can do without stopping. Take one-third to one-half of that number and do that many sit-ups, push-ups, and pull-ups as a set three times. Rest a minute or two between each set.

Some strength-training programs require special training techniques such as alternating body parts so muscles can get the rest they need. For your training program, you can do sit-ups, push-ups, and pull-ups as many as four to six days each week, or each day that you do your aerobic exercise. Make sure that you rest about two minutes between each set of exercises. Breathe out (exhale) when you exert yourself such as in the pulling position of a pull-up or the pushing portion of the push-up.

As your training progresses, you will notice increased strength. You can keep a progress record by testing yourself

Remember to avoid "bouncing" when counting how many sit-ups you can do.

every week. Use the results from the second and fourth weeks to gauge your overall progress and to decide whether your exercise sets should be increased.

For example, after the first two weeks when you test yourself again, you should also see how many pull-ups and push-ups you can do. If you can do more than you did the first time, increase the number of push-ups and pull-ups each time you exercise. As you get stronger, you need to do a greater number of repetitions and sets to continue to increase muscular strength. Once you achieve the strength you want to have, you can maintain it by doing your exercises just two to three times a week.

Weight training routines are built around repetitions and sets. A repetition is a series of a single exercise. A set is a group of repetitions of that exercise. For example, to complete two sets of 15 repetitions for the chest/bench press, you must do the chest/bench press 15 times in a row to complete one set, rest, and then do the chest/bench press another 15 times in a row to complete your second set.

Flexibility

Flexibility is defined as a joint's range of motion. The more a joint can move through a range of motion, the greater its flexibility. All joints in your body have some degree of flexibility. While the joints for which flexibility is most important depend on the sport or activity in which you are involved, overall good flexibility in all areas of the body is very important.

For the average person, the lower back and the legs need the most attention. Lower back pain is caused not only by weak abdominal muscles but also by tight lower back muscles and hamstrings. Lower back stretching exercises, in addition to abdominal strengthening exercises (sit-ups), will help prevent lower back problems.

Stretching exercises are also an important part of your warm-up for an aerobic exercise. Stretching helps get blood circulating into the working muscles, and warms them up to help prevent injury during an activity. Stretching is easy to learn, but there is a right way and a wrong way. Do your stretching exercises at the end of your warm-up, when your body is warmed to a light sweat, and again when you have completed your exercises. The right way is a stretch sustained about 20 to 30 seconds.

Try to focus your attention on the muscles being stretched, and relax. Do not bounce up and down or stretch past the point of pain. Stretch the muscle to the point where you feel a light tension on the muscle. As you feel the tension release, increase the stretch just a little until tension is felt again. Continue this for about 30 seconds, then rest and repeat the stretch two or three times. Breathe normally as you hold the stretch.

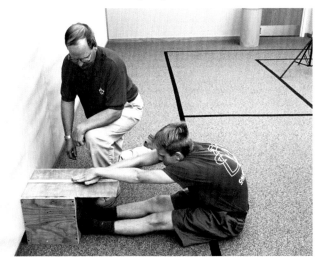

Sit and reach to measure lower-back flexibility.

The sit-and-reach test is an easy way to measure flexibility of areas such as the lower back and the back of the thighs. This test uses a special "sit-and-reach" box or similar improvised device such as a yardstick taped to a bench. This stretch works many joints and muscles, including hips, shoulders, and ankles.

To assume the starting position, remove your shoes and sit facing the sit-and-reach box. Keep your knees fully extended and flat on the floor, and place your feet against the end board. You might need to have someone gently hold your knees flat on the floor. Extend your arms forward with your hands placed on top of each other, palms down. Bend at the hips (not curling the shoulders), reach forward along the measuring scale four times, and hold your hands at the maximum position on the measuring scale for the fourth reach. Record the measurement of the fourth reach.

Making a Sit-and-Reach Device

To make the box, cut the following pieces, using any sturdy wood or ¾-inch plywood.

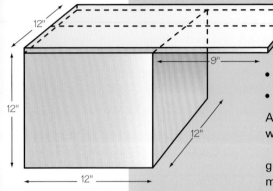

O MARK

- Four 12-by-12-inch pieces
- One 12-by-21-inch piece

Assemble the pieces using wood screws and glue.

Inscribe the top panel with gradations so that the 9-inch mark is in line with the vertical panel against which the feet will be placed. The measuring scale should extend from 0 at the front edge to 21 inches at the far end. You may choose to simply tape a yardstick to the top panel.

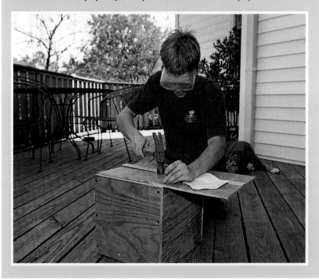

As an alternative to the sit-and-reach box, tape a yardstick to the top of a bench. Or, tape a yardstick to the edge of a bench laid on its side so that the seat is the panel against which the feet are placed. Make sure to mount the yardstick so that the 9-inch mark is in line with the panel against which the feet are placed.

Body Composition

Body composition is the proportion of your body that is fat or muscle. It normally is given as a percentage of body fat. For example, if you weigh 120 pounds and have 15 percent body fat, then you have 18 pounds of fat on your body.

A certain amount of fat is necessary to sustain life. This essential fat is located in your bones, in your nervous system, and around your internal organs. Too much fat can lead to obesity, diabetes, and cardiovascular diseases.

Typically, height and weight tables are used to decide if you are the right weight according to your age and height. These can be highly misleading because it is possible to be light in weight but technically obese. It is also possible to be lean and muscular but heavy. Knowing your body-fat composition is more important than knowing your weight.

You can measure body composition several ways. Many health-care professionals have special equipment that can quickly calculate body fat percentages and other body composition measurements.

With a tape measure, you can easily take measurements of several places, such as thighs, arms, abdomen, shoulders, and chest. Take the same measurements once a month. These numbers will not tell you your body fat percentage, but they can be used to monitor the progress of your exercise and nutrition program.

Weight control, or body composition management, is one benefit of aerobic exercises. Exercise uses calories from the foods you eat and from fat stores to provide energy for your muscles. If you are concerned about being overweight, remember that many young people who are overweight can benefit from reducing body fat while maintaining or only slightly reducing overall body mass.

Body measurements can help you check the progress of your exercise and nutrition program.

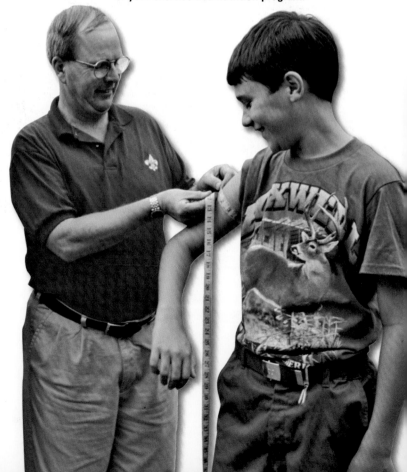

When you exercise to lose fat, low-intensity exercise for longer periods (such as lap swimming or jogging) is always best. In resistance training (such as weight lifting) to gain muscle tone, use lighter weights and increase the number of sets and repetitions (again, low intensity and longer duration). Be sure your routine includes eating the right foods in reasonable quantity.

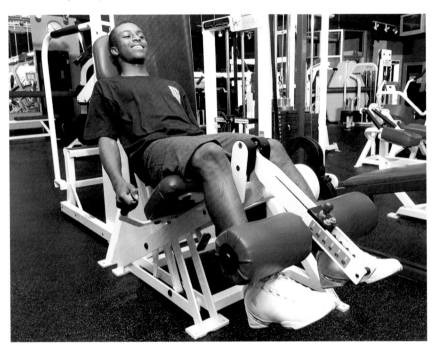

Weight control is a slow process. You cannot expect to take off quickly the fat that has built up over time. When fat needs to be lost, a one- to two-pound-per-week loss is best. This is an average rate. Some weeks you may not experience any fat loss, and other weeks, more. Rapid fat and weight loss is not recommended.

Just as you would see a physician for health and medical problems, professionals are available to give exercise and nutrition guidance. Exercise physiologists and registered dietitians from a nearby college or university usually are more than willing to meet with you or your entire troop.

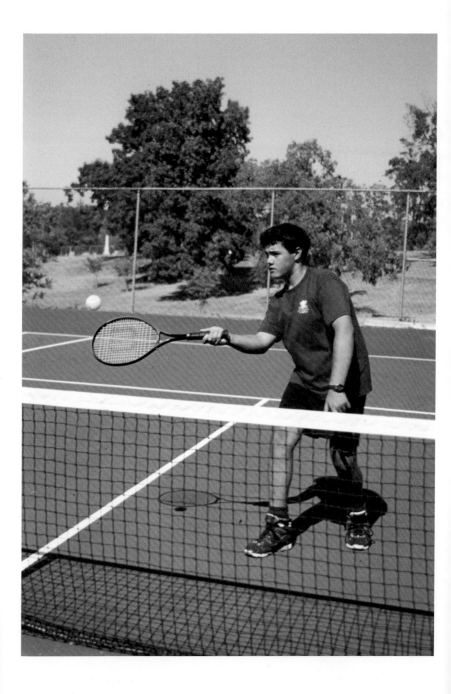

Creating a Personal Exercise Program

Regular exercise may be the single most important thing you can do to live a long and healthy life. Studies of people who live to great age—into their 90s and beyond—show that these people have at least one thing in common: regular exercise. There is a great deal more variation in other habits such as diet. While exercise has a wide variety of benefits, the most remarkable are the prevention of heart disease and the strengthening of bones.

Exercise Records

Remember that an important part of healthy exercise is the discipline of staying on a regular program. To help with this discipline, keep an accurate record of your fitness program. (This is also a merit badge requirement.) Your exercise log should record the date, describe the activity, and show the comparative measurement (number of repetitions, time, distance, number of sets, and so forth).

Keep an accurate
record of your
fitness program.

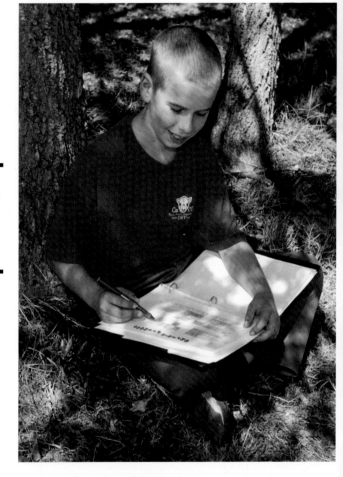

Two forms are included here for your personal record, or
you can create your own forms. On the Exercise Log, describe
your planned exercises in the left column and then simply check
off each item completed on the indicated dates. You will need
a copy of the form for each two-week period. On the Exercise
Journal, enter a daily description of your activity with one journal page for each week. Use either the log or journal format
for your daily record.

Exercise Log

Exercise Description	Week ___							Week ___							Week ___						
	Su	M	T	W	Th	F	Sa	Su	M	T	W	Th	F	Sa	Su	M	T	W	Th	F	Sa

Exercise Journal

Week _____

Date	Description of Activity

The Connection Between Good Health and Exercise

People who exercise regularly are less likely to be overweight because exercise burns up calories. Blood pressure is reduced by exercise. In fact, the combination of exercise and weight reduction often allows people with hypertension (high blood pressure) to control their blood pressure without the use of medication. This control may be better than was possible with drugs.

It is common for smokers to quit smoking as they begin exercise programs. Research has shown that active joggers have lower total cholesterol than men of the same age who do not run. There is no substitute for exercise when it comes to protecting your heart.

Without sufficient exercise, bones lose their calcium and become brittle. This demineralization of bones has been documented in astronauts returning from space, where the lack of gravity robs activity of its exercise value. Weak and brittle bones, caused by lack of exercise, are common in the elderly. Strong bones contribute to personal fitness by keeping an active person energetic.

Types of Exercise

People who exercise regularly feel and look younger than those who do not. Improvements in muscle tone and circulation undoubtedly contribute to freedom from fatigue and the feeling of well-being that the physically fit enjoy.

The connection between being in good shape and being productive is also a powerful one. Research has shown that healthy people are more productive and efficient than those who are not healthy.

For people who are limited by choice or circumstances to one form of exercise, a full-body exercise is strongly recommended. In full-body exercise, all muscles and joints are moved and flexed. Such forms of exercise include brisk walking, running, cycling, rowing, and swimming.

Walking, particularly brisk "power walks" of several miles on a daily basis, can give many of the same benefits as running without most of the injury risks. Walking can also be done at any age without special equipment or facilities. Cycling, too, matches and even enhances the health benefits of running by eliminating impact stress. However, it does have a relatively high injury rate and requires special equipment.

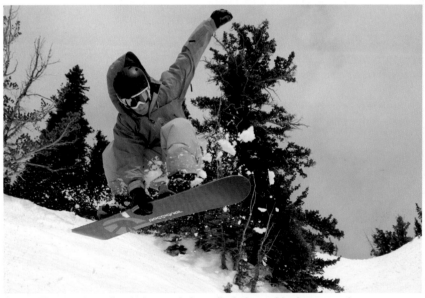

Sports like snowboarding help people keep fit during cold winter months.

Rowing and swimming are to some degree superior to other types of full-body exercise because both the upper and lower body are fully involved (assuming you are rowing a sliding-seat craft or simulator). The injury rates for rowing and swimming exercise are very low, and there is no impact stress in either activity. Joint stress is further reduced in swimming by the buoyancy effect of water immersion. But rowing requires relatively expensive special equipment, and swimming requires access to a suitable, safe facility.

Many sports incorporate full-body exercise such as tennis, golf (if you walk the course), and team sports such as soccer or basketball. The fun and competition of sports add further incentive for healthy exercise. In terms of healthy lifestyle, every person should choose a form of exercise or sport that can be pursued and enjoyed for a lifetime. Among the many benefits will be a significantly healthier—and longer—life.

Water sports are popular during the long, hot days of summer.

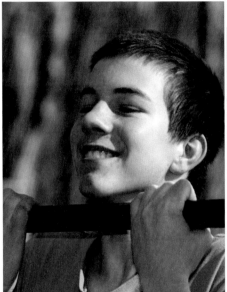

Test yourself to see your physical fitness progress.

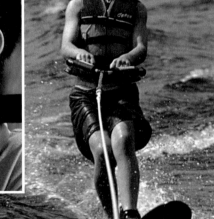

Physical Fitness Tests

It is important to know your current level of fitness to create the best possible exercise program for you. The following tests will help you measure your physical fitness. You will also use these tests to fulfill your merit badge requirements. Each test must be administered by, or under the supervision of, your merit badge counselor.

Aerobic Fitness Test

Record your performance on one of the following tests:

1. Run/walk as far as you can and as fast as you can in nine minutes.

OR

2. Run/walk 1 mile as fast as you can.

Flexibility Test

Using a sit-and-reach box constructed according to specifications in this merit badge pamphlet, make four repetitions and record the fourth reach. This last reach must be held steady for 15 seconds to qualify. (Remember to keep your knees down.)

Strength Tests

Record your performance on all three tests.

1. *Sit-ups*—Record the number of sit-ups done correctly in 60 seconds. The sit-ups must be done in the form explained and illustrated in the merit badge pamphlet.

2. *Pull-ups*—Record the total number of pull-ups completed correctly in 60 seconds. Be consistent with the procedures presented in the merit badge pamphlet.

3. *Push-ups*—Record the total number of push-ups completed correctly in 60 seconds. Be consistent with the procedures presented in the merit badge pamphlet.

Pull-Ups
Begin the exercise hanging from the bar with arms fully extended and hands on the bar, palms forward and directly above the shoulders. Pull up until you can touch the top of the bar with the bottom of your outstretched chin.

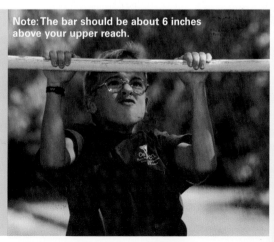

Note: The bar should be about 6 inches above your upper reach.

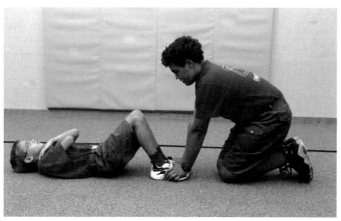

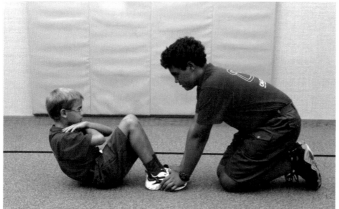

Sit-Ups

To assume the starting position, lie on your back with knees flexed, feet on the floor, and heels between 12 and 18 inches from the buttocks. The arms are crossed on the chest with the hands on the opposite shoulders. The feet are held by a partner to keep them on the floor. Curl to the sitting position until the elbows touch the thighs. Arms must remain on the chest and chin tucked on the chest. Return to the starting position, shoulder blades touching the floor.

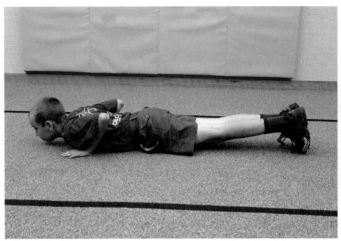

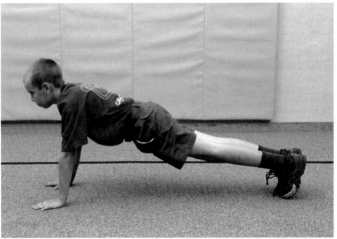

Push-Ups

Begin in a prone position on the floor with the palms flat on the floor under the shoulders. The feet are flexed up with the ball of the foot and the toes on the floor. Push up by fully extending the arms. Try not to lock the elbows. The shoulders, hips, and legs should remain in a straight line from the heels to the head.

Body Composition Test

Have your parent, counselor, or other adult take and record the following measurements.

1. Circumference of the right upper arm midway between the shoulder and the elbow with the arm hanging naturally, and not flexed

2. Shoulders with arms hanging by placing the tape measure 2 inches below the top of the shoulders around the arms, chest, and back after breath expiration

3. Chest by placing the tape under the arms and around the chest and back at the nipple line after breath expiration

4. Abdomen circumference at the navel level (relaxed)

5. Circumference of the right thigh midway between the hip and knee, and not flexed

If possible, have the same person take these measurements whenever you are ready to be remeasured to chart your progress.

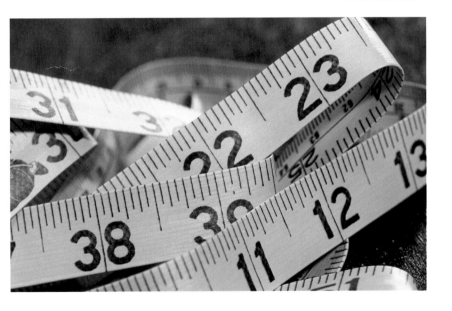

Fitness Measurements

Aerobic Fitness	Start	2nd Week	4th Week	6th Week	8th Week	10th Week	12th Week	Goal
9-Minute Run/Walk (Yards completed)								
1-Mile Run/Walk (In minutes and seconds)								

You may choose either the nine-minute run/walk for distance OR the 1-mile run/walk for time. You may also do both for extra experience and benefit.

Strength	Start	2nd Week	4th Week	6th Week	8th Week	10th Week	12th Week	Goal
Sit-Ups								
Push-Ups								
Pull-Ups								

You must do the sit-ups exercise and one other (either push-ups or pull-ups). You may also do all three for extra experience and benefit. (Measurements should be in numbers and repetitions.)

Flexibility	Start	2nd Week	4th Week	6th Week	8th Week	10th Week	12th Week	Goal
Reach (In centimeters)								

Body Composition	Start	2nd Week	4th Week	6th Week	8th Week	10th Week	12th Week	Goal
Right Arm Circumference								
Shoulder Circumference								
Chest Circumference								
Abdomen Circumference								
Right Thigh Circumference								

Remember that each set of measurements should be taken by the same adult, if possible. Measurements should be in inches.

Your Fitness Program

Your comprehensive fitness program should be individualized to your own starting level based on your physical fitness test scores and personal goals or objectives. Whatever your starting level, exercise activity, and fitness objectives, your comprehensive program should include these five elements:

1. Warm-up
2. Aerobic exercises
3. Strength exercises
4. Flexibility exercises
5. Cool-down

Warm-Up

The warm-up routine should be several minutes of low-intensity movement and then some muscle stretching. For example, you could do a light jog or run in place for two to three minutes; skip rope at a moderate pace for one to two minutes; walk briskly for three to five minutes; or swim a crawl or trudgen stroke at slow to medium speed for 50 to 100 yards. This low-intensity exercise should then be followed by two to three minutes of stretching exercises.

Aerobic Exercises

A good aerobic routine begins with some form of wind sprints (short duration, full-speed exertion) repeated three to five times with one to three minutes of rest intervals in between. For example, running a 50-yard dash, resting three minutes, then repeating the cycle two more times would be a good wind sprint set for your first week.

A 25-yard dash on a competitive swimming stroke (front crawl, back crawl, breaststroke, or butterfly) repeated three times with two to three minutes of rest intervals would also be a good wind sprint set using swimming skills. Similar routines could use jumping rope, skating, calisthenics, or any high-aerobic activity.

Follow the wind sprints, after a three- to five-minute rest, with a mid-distance exercise—a 600-yard run or a 400-yard swim, for example. As your aerobic performance improves, increase your number of sprints and the length of your mid-distance exercise.

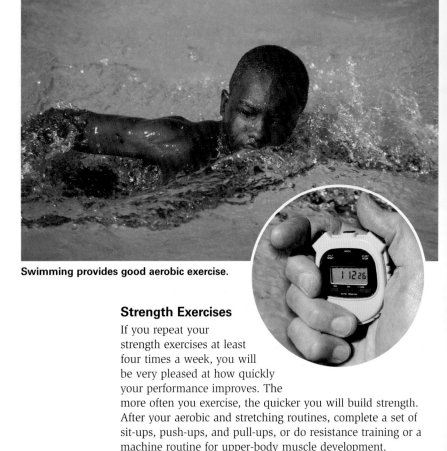

Swimming provides good aerobic exercise.

Strength Exercises

If you repeat your strength exercises at least four times a week, you will be very pleased at how quickly your performance improves. The more often you exercise, the quicker you will build strength. After your aerobic and stretching routines, complete a set of sit-ups, push-ups, and pull-ups, or do resistance training or a machine routine for upper-body muscle development.

Always try to improve at least a little on your previous number of repetitions. You may want to do your exercises in several sets with a few minutes of rest between sets. (For example, you could do a set of 15 push-ups, rest; do 10 push-ups, rest; and do five push-ups.)

Remember to keep a log of your activity. Doing this will remind you to rest your muscles for at least a day after a strength-training workout before working the same muscles again.

Flexibility Exercises

Follow your strength exercises with a flexibility workout.

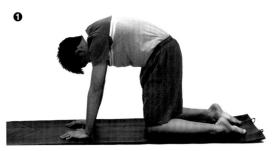

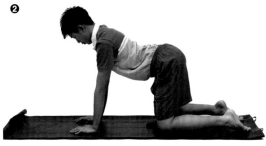

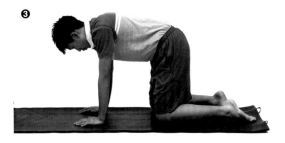

Cats and Camels

Step 1—Get on your hands and knees as shown, with your hands and knees a shoulder's width apart.

Step 2—Slowly arch your back upward, toward the ceiling, then lower it toward the floor.

Step 3—Straighten your back to a comfortable position. Slowly repeat steps 1 through 3, five times.

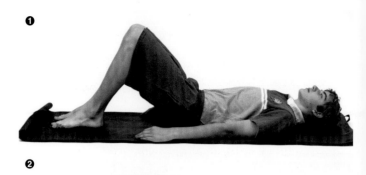

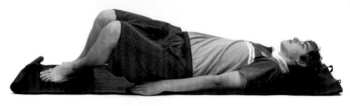

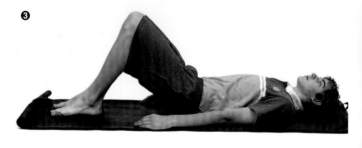

Lower Trunk Rotations

Step 1—Lie flat on your back with your knees bent as shown.

Step 2—Keep your knees together and slowly lower them to the left. Hold this position for 10 to 15 seconds.

Step 3—Raise your knees back to the starting position, then slowly lower your knees to the right and hold this position for 10 to 15 seconds.

Repeat steps 1 through 3, three times on each side.

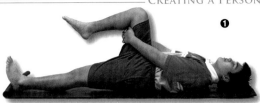

Hamstring Stretch

Step 1—Lie flat on your back and extend one knee toward your head, as shown, with your hands clasped together at the back of your knee.

Step 2—Slowly lift your foot upward, toward the ceiling, until you feel a stretch in the back side of your thigh or calf. Hold this position for 15 to 20 seconds. (To obtain a better stretch, use a towel or belt wrapped around your foot to pull with your hands and arms.)

Step 3—Slowly lower your leg and return to the starting position. Repeat steps 1 through 3, three times for each leg.

Cool-Down

After your last exercise, get up and walk around or take a casual swim. If you are walking, move your arms back and forth, then up and down. Do not simply roll over and play dead after your last exercise. The cool-down routine helps prevent muscle cramps and enhances the aerobic and flexibility benefits of your exercise. If you simply "play dead," when you do try to get up you may feel light-headed or dizzy and risk fainting or nausea.

After your cool-down exercises, check your pulse for regular beat.

Sample Program

Refer to the Sample Physical Fitness Program starting later in this chapter. This program is for an already physically active Scout who is fairly aggressive about the benefits he wants to achieve. He also has access to a swimming pool and some special exercise equipment.

For variety, the sample program has several warm-up and exercise options. You can include options or alternative routines in your program, or choose one specific routine. Remember to consider access and convenience in making these selections.

If you are going swimming, biking, skating, or whatever your routine, be sure to follow all safety rules and requirements. Do not attempt to use weights or other special equipment without getting instruction on the safe use of this equipment from a coach, instructor, or experienced user.

Now, using the sample program as a model, list your personal fitness test results and personal goals to plan your own 12-week fitness program. Begin by filling in the last column (Goals) on your fitness measurement sheet. Decide what you want to achieve on each of the aerobic, flexibility, and strength measurements. Be realistic, but challenge yourself to make a substantial improvement on each measure. Then figure out what routines will get you from your starting measurements to your goals. Plan your fitness program accordingly. You may want to adjust and revise your program every week or two as you progress. Be sure that your program is reviewed and approved by your counselor before you begin the exercises.

Sample Physical Fitness Program

Warm-Up Routine
(Practiced before each aerobic or strength routine)

1. Do ONE of the following:
    a. Jog or run in place two to three minutes.
    b. Do an easy rope skip for one to two minutes.
    c. Walk briskly for three to five minutes.
    d. Swim an easy stroke at a slow speed for 100 yards.
2. Do stretching exercises for three to five minutes.

Aerobic Routine
(Two or three times per week; alternate with the strength routine. The distance, repetitions, and rest intervals should be reviewed and adjusted weekly as your performance improves.)

1. Wind sprints:

    Running distance _____ Repetitions _____ Rest time _____

    Swimming distance _____ Repetitions _____ Rest time _____

2. Mid-distance workout (best time). Do ONE of the following:

    a. 600-yard run   b. 400-yard swim

Strength Routine
(Two or three times per week; alternate with aerobic routine; weights, repetitions, and rest intervals to be reviewed and adjusted weekly, as appropriate)

Weight lifting:

1. Press:
   Weight _____ Repetitions _____ Sets _____ Rest time _____

2. Curls:
   Weight _____ Repetitions _____ Sets _____ Rest time _____

3. Bench press:
   Weight _____ Repetitions _____ Sets _____ Rest time _____

4. Squats:
   Weight _____ Repetitions _____ Sets _____ Rest time _____

Flexibility Routine
(Five times per week)

1. Hamstring stretch. Lie flat; extend one knee toward the head, with hands clasped together behind the knee. Slowly lift the foot upward, hold 15–20 seconds, then slowly lower back to the starting position. Repeat with the other leg. Do three repetitions.

2. Lower trunk rotations. Lie flat with knees slightly bent. Keep the knees together and slowly lower them to the left; hold 10–15 seconds. Raise the knees back to the starting position, then slowly lower the knees to the right; hold 10–15 seconds. Do three repetitions.

3. Cats and camels. Get on hands and knees, with hands and knees a shoulder's width apart. Slowly arch the back upward, then lower it toward the floor. Straighten the back to a comfortable position. Do five repetitions.

Cool-Down
(Five-minute "walk-and-talk" after each aerobic or strength routine)

Do not neglect the cool-down period, which helps prevent muscle cramps after exercise and enhances the benefits of your physical fitness program.

Analyzing Your Record

After your 12th week, compare your last measurements and test performance to your first. Requirement 8 says that you must show improvement on the aerobic, flexibility, and muscular strength tests. If you have shortened your time for the mile run or doubled your number of pull-ups, the *quantity* of your performance has improved. But think also about your fitness *quality:*

- What is your recovery time after strenuous exercise? (How long does it take for your heart rate to return to its normal, resting rate?)

- What changes have occurred in your overall stamina and endurance?

- Are you more or less sleepy during the day?

- Have your eating habits changed?

- Do you enjoy participating in physical activities?

Also, compare your body composition measurements:

- Have you added muscle mass or reduced your volume of body fat?

- How do your chest and stomach measurements relate after 12 weeks of exercise? Is the ratio of these two measurements different from your preprogram measurements? If you have been conscientious in pursuing your program, the difference between your chest and stomach measurements (chest measurement minus stomach measurement) should have changed.

- Do you think you look and feel different? If you feel different, describe and explain this difference to your counselor.

Ask yourself what this experience has taught you about commitment and self-discipline. Think about what you have learned about your body's adaptability and response to activity.

Many fitness experts today believe that, on average, today's young people are significantly less physically fit than previous generations. The tables that follow reflect test performance for American young people.

Find your percentile level on the various measurements. How do you compare on both your beginning and final scores? How far up the scale did you progress after only three months of regular exercise?

In terms of your own goals, what was your success? Did you achieve the performance level you targeted for each of the aerobic, endurance, flexibility, and strength measurements? If not, your goals may have been unrealistic or your fitness program may not have been sufficiently challenging. Or maybe you simply did not make the full effort that you could have.

Based on your experience, what would you do differently in designing another fitness program for yourself? Will personal fitness be a priority for you in the future? If so, what will you do to keep fit?

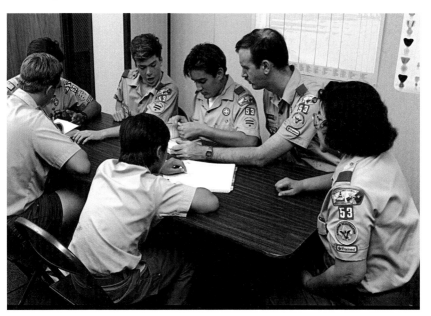

Table 1. Percentile Norms for the 1-Mile Run* for Boys Ages 10 to 18

Age	10	11	12	13	14	15	16	17+
Percentile	Time (In minutes and seconds)							
99	6:25	6:04	5:40	5:44	5:36	5:44	5:40	5:41
95	6:56	6:50	6:27	6:11	5:51	6:01	5:48	6:01
90	7:26	7:19	6:44	6:22	6:05	6:08	6:02	6:13
85	7:40	7:30	6:57	6:33	6:13	6:18	6:12	6:28
80	7:57	7:48	7:12	6:42	6:21	6:29	6:22	6:30
75	8:10	8:00	7:24	6:52	6:36	6:35	6:28	6:36
70	8:23	8:08	7:37	7:00	6:41	6:42	6:41	6:42
65	8:34	8:21	7:48	7:06	6:48	6:56	6:47	6:57
60	8:49	8:39	7:59	7:14	6:54	7:02	6:53	7:07
55	9:03	8:56	8:08	7:20	7:01	7:07	7:03	7:15
50	9:19	9:06	8:20	7:27	7:10	7:14	7:11	7:25
45	9:34	9:25	8:34	7:40	7:15	7:23	7:19	7:30
40	9:45	9:46	8:51	7:51	7:24	7:30	7:27	7:45
35	10:10	10:10	9:10	8:02	7:34	7:41	7:40	7:58
30	10:38	10:40	9:30	8:24	7:54	7:52	7:51	8:06
25	11:05	11:31	10:00	8:35	8:02	8:04	8:07	8:26
20	11:31	12:02	10:42	8:50	8:15	8:26	8:41	8:38
15	12:11	12:40	11:20	9:09	8:43	8:48	9:10	9:05
10	13:00	13:37	12:07	9:39	9:30	9:25	9:52	10:37
5	14:28	15:25	13:41	10:23	10:32	10:37	10:40	10:56

*Health-Related Physical Fitness Test from the American Alliance for Health, Physical Education, Recreation and Dance

Table 2. Percentile Norms for the 9-Minute Run* for Boys Ages 10 to 18

Age	10	11	12	13	14	15	16	17+
Percentile	Distance (In yards)							
99	2,520	2,520	2,880	2,615	2,686	2,757	2,828	2,899
95	2,250	2,250	2,400	2,402	2,473	2,544	2,615	2,615
90	2,120	2,109	2,175	2,320	2,391	2,462	2,533	2,604
85	2,013	2,025	2,042	2,213	2,284	2,384	2,455	2,526
80	1,950	1,970	2,000	2,150	2,221	2,292	2,363	2,434
75	1,910	1,925	1,975	2,096	2,167	2,238	2,309	2,380
70	1,859	1,890	1,900	2,049	2,120	2,191	2,262	2,333
65	1,810	1,860	1,860	2,008	2,079	2,150	2,221	2,292
60	1,780	1,808	1,810	1,964	2,035	2,106	2,177	2,248
55	1,725	1,770	1,790	1,926	1,997	2,068	2,139	2,210
50	1,690	1,725	1,760	1,885	1,956	2,027	2,098	2,169
45	1,633	1,690	1,740	1,844	1,915	1,986	2,057	2,128
40	1,600	1,640	1,680	1,806	1,877	1,948	2,019	2,090
35	1,584	1,600	1,620	1,762	1,833	1,904	1,975	2,046
30	1,536	1,575	1,590	1,721	1,792	1,863	1,934	2,005
25	1,487	1,540	1,500	1,674	1,745	1,816	1,887	1,958
20	1,420	1,440	1,450	1,620	1,691	1,762	1,833	1,904
15	1,356	1,390	1,356	1,557	1,628	1,699	1,770	1,841
10	1,250	1,275	1,300	1,450	1,521	1,592	1,663	1,734
5	1,110	1,170	1,000	1,368	1,439	1,510	1,581	1,652

*Health-Related Physical Fitness Test from the American Alliance for Health, Physical Education, Recreation and Dance

Table 3. Percentile Norms for the Sit and Reach*
for Boys Ages 10 to 18

Age	10	11	12	13	14	15	16	17+
Percentile	**Reaches (In centimeters)**							
99	37	38	52	41	43	47	45	48
95	33	34	35	36	39	41	42	45
90	31	32	32	34	37	39	40	43
85	30	31	31	33	36	37	38	41
80	29	30	30	32	34	36	37	40
75	28	29	29	30	33	34	36	40
70	28	28	29	29	31	33	35	38
65	22	27	28	28	30	32	34	37
60	26	26	27	27	30	32	32	36
55	26	26	27	27	29	31	31	35
50	25	25	26	26	28	30	30	34
45	24	24	25	25	27	29	29	33
40	23	23	24	24	26	28	28	32
35	22	23	23	23	25	27	27	31
30	21	33	33	33	34	26	26	30
25	20	21	21	20	23	24	25	28
20	19	20	20	19	22	23	23	26
15	18	18	18	18	21	22	21	25
10	17	16	16	15	18	19	18	23
5	12	12	13	12	15	13	11	15

*Health-Related Physical Fitness Test from the American Alliance for Health, Physical Education, Recreation and Dance

Table 4. Percentile Norms for Sit-Ups*
for Boys Ages 10 to 18

Age	10	11	12	13	14	15	16	17+
Percentile	Number of Sit-Ups							
99	59	61	68	70	70	69	70	65
95	50	51	56	58	59	59	61	62
90	47	48	52	54	54	55	59	59
85	44	46	50	52	52	52	55	59
80	42	44	48	50	51	50	53	54
75	40	42	46	48	49	49	51	52
70	39	41	45	46	48	48	50	51
65	37	40	43	45	46	47	49	50
60	36	39	42	44	45	46	47	49
55	35	38	40	42	44	45	46	48
50	34	37	39	41	42	44	45	46
45	33	35	38	40	41	42	44	45
40	31	34	36	39	40	41	42	44
35	30	33	35	38	39	40	40	43
30	29	31	33	36	38	39	39	40
25	27	30	31	35	36	38	38	38
20	25	28	30	33	35	36	35	37
15	23	26	28	31	33	34	33	34
10	19	23	25	29	31	31	30	31
5	15	17	19	25	27	28	28	25

*Health-Related Physical Fitness Test from the American Alliance for Health, Physical Education, Recreation and Dance

Careers in Personal Fitness

There are many exciting careers in the field of personal fitness.

Personal trainers should have written policies explaining their services, costs, cancellations, length of contract, and emergency procedures. They should also require a medical clearance form to be completed before they work with individual clients.

Exercise Physiologist

An exercise physiologist can prescribe exercise programs for cardiac and pulmonary patients referred by physicians. They teach people about the benefits of exercise. Exercise physiologists also evaluate cardiovascular and metabolic effects in people, and help active athletes improve and maintain their health and athletic performance.

Most exercise physiologists hold a master's degree in exercise science and have taken numerous courses in human anatomy and physiology, chemistry, biomechanics, kinesiology, exercise testing and prescription, and sports nutrition. An internship is part of the curriculum.

Colleges and universities, rehabilitation clinics, hospitals, sports and athletic programs, and health/fitness facilities hire exercise physiologists. They frequently serve as sports and wellness program instructors and directors, teachers, or academic researchers.

Personal Trainer

A qualified personal trainer has an education in physiology, health promotion, athletic training, kinesiology, or a similar field. They should hold first-aid and CPR certifications.

Once considered a luxury for wealthy people who needed help keeping up with an exercise routine, personal training has undergone an overall transformation in the past several years, emerging as one of the fastest-growing professions of this decade.

Today, fitness professionals have an in-depth knowledge of anatomy and physiology. Some are even qualified in rehabilitation, nutrition, psychology, and fitness therapies, as well as strength, conditioning, and flexibility programs.

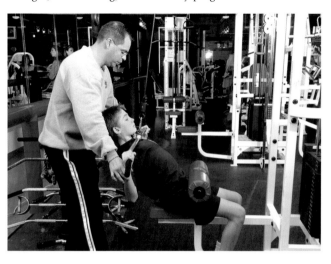

Good trainers have excellent communication skills and can motivate, lead, instruct, and guide their clients to make better decisions regarding their own personal fitness. Some courses can be studied and passed in as little as 25 hours of study, while others can take three to four years to complete.

Dietician or Nutritionist

To become a dietician, you need a four-year degree in dietetics or nutrition with a nine- to 12-month internship or completion of an undergraduate program that combines classroom and clinical experience.

A certified nutritionist (CN) or certified clinical nutritionist (CCN) has had extensive education and training in nutrition science and has met national testing standards. Both CNs and CCNs work with clients to figure out individual nutritional needs and develop individual nutrition plans. They educate, advise, counsel, monitor, and provide support to their clients. Doctors often refer their patients to nutritionists for dietary counseling.

A certified nutritionist must earn a bachelor of science or higher degree in nutrition science from an accredited college or formal training program that is recognized by state licensing agencies. Certified nutritionists must also complete a series of exams required by the National Institute of Nutritional Education.

A certified clinical nutritionist must have received a graduate degree in a health-care field or, if he or she holds only a bachelor's degree, must also complete 900 hours of medical and clinical nutrition internship. Certified clinical nutritionists are then qualified to take case histories and use various tests and observations to assess an individual's nutritional needs.

Most states require a license for professional dietitians but the situation is not nearly as clear for nutritionists. The Society of Certified Nutritionists (SCN) is working to establish national standards of practice in that field.

Coaches and Scouts

As a coach, you will need to work hard to instill both motivation and determination in your players, even when your athletes go through plateau periods when they cannot seem to beat their own best time or are on a losing streak. Coaches help evaluate athletes' personal strengths and weaknesses to help them improve their performance.

Coaches are responsible for the training and development of athletes and sports teams. Scouts conduct searches for talented players for various team sports on the college and professional levels.

For high school coaching jobs, schools normally hire teachers willing to work at coaching part-time. If you feel you can help motivate athletes, plan and manage practice sessions, instruct groups or individuals in the basics of sports, and find and recruit athletes for college-level or professional leagues, and if you like to travel, this may be the career for you.

Many scouts played a sport at the college or professional level, which helps them pick out promising players from the crowd.

To get into the coaching field, you will need to earn a teaching degree in secondary education or a physical education teaching degree.

Certified Athletic Trainers

A certified athletic trainer is a medical expert in preventing, recognizing, managing, and rehabilitating injuries that result from physical activity. As part of a complete health-care team, the certified athletic trainer works under the direction of a licensed physician and in cooperation with other health-care professionals, athletic administrators, coaches, and parents. A certified athletic trainer's day may include preparing athletes for practice or competition, including taping, bandaging and bracing; evaluating injuries to determine their management and possible referral to another health-care practitioner; and developing treatment and rehabilitation programs.

Physical therapists not only create treatment plans and help patients carry them out, but they also serve as teachers and coaches, inspiring patients to lead more complete lives.

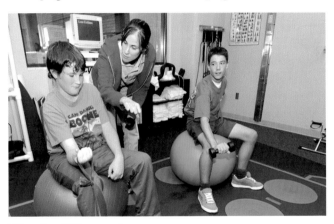

Physical Therapists

People who have trouble using their muscles need the help of a physical therapist. Elderly people recovering from knee-replacement surgery, injured athletes, children with muscular diseases and birth defects, and young people with brain disorders are all potential clients for physical therapists.

These health professionals use exercises and many other techniques to get their patients moving. They also teach them how to get around using crutches and wheelchairs, and using prosthetic limbs.

You need an advanced degree from an accredited four-year college or university and a passing score on a state-licensing exam to become a physical therapist. You should be good at communication skills, and being physically strong can help you in your career as well.

The Scout Oath and the Scout Law

As part of your personal fitness program, demonstrate Scout spirit by living the Scout Oath and Scout Law in your everyday life.

The Scout Oath

On my honor I will do my best
To do my duty to God and my country
and to obey the Scout Law;
To help other people at all times;
To keep myself physically strong,
mentally awake, and morally straight.

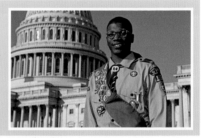

The Meaning of the Scout Oath

Before you pledge yourself to any oath or promise, you must know what it means.

On my honor . . .

By giving your word, you are promising to be guided by the ideals of the Scout Oath.

. . . I will do my best . . .

Try hard to live up to the points of the Scout Oath. Measure your achievements against your own high standards and do not be influenced by peer pressure or what other people do.

. . .To do my duty to God . . .

Your family and religious leaders teach you about God and the ways you can serve. You do your duty to God by following the wisdom of those teachings every day and by respecting and defending the rights of others to practice their own beliefs.

. . . and my country . . .

Help keep the United States a strong and fair nation by learning about our system of government and your responsibilities as a citizen and future voter.

The United States is made up of countless families and communities. When you work to improve your community and your home, you are serving your country. Natural resources are another important part of this country's heritage worthy of your efforts to understand, protect, and use wisely. What you do can make a real difference.

. . . and to obey the Scout Law; . . .

The 12 points of the Scout Law are guidelines that can lead you toward wise choices. When you obey the Scout Law, other people will respect you for the way you live, and you will respect yourself.

. . . To help other people at all times; . . .

There are many people who need you. Your cheerful smile and helping hand will ease the burden of many who need assistance. By helping out whenever possible, you are doing your part to make this a better world.

. . . To keep myself physically strong, . . .

Take care of your body so that it will serve you well for an entire lifetime. That means eating nutritious foods, getting enough sleep, and exercising regularly to build strength and endurance. It also means avoiding harmful drugs, alcohol, tobacco, and anything else that can harm your health.

. . . mentally awake, . . .

Develop your mind both in the classroom and outside of school. Be curious about everything around you, and work hard to make the most of your abilities. With an inquiring attitude and the willingness to ask questions, you can learn much about the exciting world around you and your role in it.

. . . and morally straight.

To be a person of strong character, your relationships with others should be honest and open. You should respect and defend the rights of all people. Be clean in your speech and actions, and remain faithful in your religious beliefs. The values you practice as a Scout will help you shape a life of virtue.

The Meaning of the Scout Law

The Scout Law is the foundation of Scouting. It is expressed in just 12 simple points, but the standards they set for you are high. Use the Scout Law to guide your actions when you are alone and as a member of your family, community, and nation. The Scout Law will show you how to live as a boy and as a man.

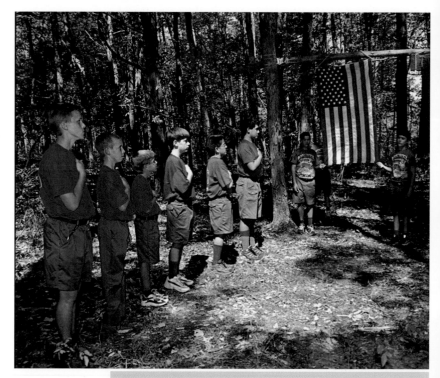

The Scout Law

A Scout is trustworthy, loyal, helpful, friendly, courteous, kind, obedient, cheerful, thrifty, brave, clean, and reverent.

A Scout is **trustworthy.** A Scout tells the truth. He is honest, and he keeps his promises. People can depend on him.

A Scout is **loyal.** A Scout is true to his family, friends, Scout leaders, school, and nation.

A Scout is **helpful.** A Scout cares about other people. He willingly volunteers to help others without expecting payment or reward.

A Scout is **friendly.** A Scout is a friend to all. He is a brother to other Scouts. He offers his friendship to people of all races and nations, and respects them even if their beliefs and customs differ from his own.

A Scout is **courteous.** A Scout is polite to everyone regardless of age or position. He knows that using good manners makes it easier for people to get along.

A Scout is **kind.** A Scout knows there is strength in being gentle. He treats others as he wants to be treated. Without good reason, he does not harm or kill any living thing.

A Scout is **obedient**. A Scout follows the rules of his family, school, and troop. He obeys the laws of his community and country. If he thinks these rules and laws are unfair, he tries to have them changed in an orderly manner rather than disobeying them.

A Scout is **cheerful.** A Scout looks for the bright side of life. He cheerfully does tasks that come his way. He tries to make others happy.

A Scout is **thrifty.** A Scout works to pay his way and to help others. He saves for the future. He protects and conserves natural resources. He carefully uses time and property.

A Scout is **brave.** A Scout can face danger although he is afraid. He has the courage to stand for what he thinks is right even if others laugh at him or threaten him.

A Scout is **clean.** A Scout keeps his body and mind fit. He chooses the company of those who live by high standards. He helps keep his home and community clean.

A Scout is **reverent.** A Scout is reverent toward God. He is faithful in his religious duties. He respects the beliefs of others.

Personal Fitness Resources

Scouting Literature

Boy Scout Journal; *Athletics, Cycling, Dentistry, Disabilities Awareness, Family Life, Public Health, Sports,* and *Swimming* merit badge pamphlets; *Boy Scout Handbook; Fieldbook*

Visit the Boy Scouts of America's official retail Web site at *http://www.scoutstuff.org* for a complete listing of all merit badge pamphlets and other helpful Scouting materials and supplies.

Diet

American Heart Association. *The American Heart Association Kids' Cookbook.* Random House, 1993.

Figtree, Dale. *Eat Smart: A Guide to Good Health for Kids.* New Win Publishing, 1997.

Drugs

Hirschfelder, Arlene B. *Kick Butts! A Kid's Action Guide to a Tobacco-Free America.* Silver Burdett Press, 1998.

Health and Fitness

Armstrong, Neil, and Joanne Welsman. *Young People and Physical Activity.* Oxford Medical Publications, Oxford University Press, 1997.

Baechle, Thomas R. *Essentials of Strength Training and Conditioning.* Human Kinetics Publishers, 1994.

Cooper, Kenneth H., with William Proctor. *Fit Kids!: The Complete Shape-Up Program From Birth Through High School.* Broadman & Holdman Publishers, 1999.

Frost, Simon. *Fitness for Young People: A Flowmotion Book: Strength, Flexibility, and Stamina Through Personal Fitness.* Sterling, 2003.

Lam, Dr. Paul. *T'ai Chi for Young People.* Wellspring Media, 2000.

Larimore, Walt, M.D., and Traci Mullins. *10 Essentials of Highly Healthy People.* Zondervan, 2003.

Lark, Liz. *Yoga: Essential Yoga Poses to Help Young People Get Fit, Supple, and Healthy.* Sterling, 2003.

Lockette, Kevin F., and Ann M. Keyes. *Conditioning with Physical Disabilities.* Human Kinetics Publishers, 1994.

Schwarzenegger, Arnold, with Charles Gaines. *Arnold's Fitness for Kids Ages 11–14: A Guide to Health, Exercise, and Nutrition.* Doubleday & Company, 1993.

Thompson, Daley, and Peter Walker. *Going for Gold: Daley Thompson's Book of Total Fitness and Body Care for Young People.* HarperCollins Publishers, 1987.

Wehman, Paul. *Life Beyond the Classroom: Transition Strategies for Young People with Disabilities.* Paul H Brookes Publishing Co., 1995.

Sports and Recreation

Glover, Bob, et al. *The Runner's Handbook: The Best-Selling Classic Fitness Guide for Beginner and Intermediate Runners.* Penguin USA, 1996.

Hayes, Larry, et al. *The Junior Golf Book.* St. Martin's Press, 1996.

Kirby, Daniel. *The ABC's of Golf.* Coyote Publishing, 1999.

Murphy, Pat, et al. *Complete Conditioning for Baseball.* Human Kinetics Publishers, 1997.

Schubert, Mark, and Heinz Kluetmeier. *Sports Illustrated Competitive Swimming: Techniques for Champions.* Sports Illustrated, 1990.

Yessis, Michael. *Sports and Fitness Success from 6 to 16.* Masters Press, 1997.

Web Sites and Organizations
Amateur-Sports.com
Web site: *http://www.amateur-sports.com*

American Dietetic Association
120 S. Riverside Plaza, Suite 2000
Chicago, IL 60606-6995
Toll-free telephone: 800-877-1600
Web site: *http://www.eatright.org*

Fit Family, Fit Kids
Centers for Disease Control and Prevention
1600 Clifton Road
Atlanta, GA 30333
Telephone: 404-639-3311
Web site: *http://www.fitfamilyfitkids.com*

Fitness for Kids
9100 Wilshire Blvd., Suite 250 W
Beverly Hills, CA 90212
Telephone: 310-275-4141
Web site: *http://www.fitnessforkids.org*

International Food Information Council Foundation
1100 Connecticut Ave. NW, Suite 430
Washington, DC 20036
Telephone: 202-296-6540
Fax: 202-296-6547
Web site: *http://ific.org*

KidsHealth
Web site: *http://www.kidshealth.org*

National Athletic Trainer's Association
2952 Stemmons Freeway
Dallas, TX 75247
Telephone: 214-637-6282
Web site: *http://www.nata.org*

Acknowledgments

The Boy Scouts of America thanks Rose Bily, a Certified Personal Trainer in Dallas, Texas, for her time, expertise, and assistance with this new edition of the *Personal Fitness* merit badge pamphlet. We are grateful to Suzanne Rocque, M.S., ATC, CSCS, head athletic trainer, University at Buffalo, State University of New York, for her assistance and input. We also appreciate Sam Coppoletti, MPT, ACCE, CSCS, clinical director and senior instructor for the Physical Therapist Assistant Program at Shawnee State University, Portsmouth, Ohio, for his assistance.

Thanks to personal trainers John Charles and Jeremy Duke of Womack's Personal Training Gym in Keller, Texas, for lending their expertise.

We appreciate the Quicklist Consulting Committee of the Association for Library Service to Children, a division of the American Library Association, for its assistance with updating the resources section of this merit badge pamphlet.

The BSA is grateful to K. Gregory Tucker, Silver Buffalo Award recipient and former chair of the BSA Health and Safety Committee (1991–98), for his leadership in revising the 1999 edition of the *Personal Fitness* merit badge pamphlet, upon which this new edition is based. Grateful acknowledgment also goes to Pat Vehrs and Jim George of Brigham Young University for their assistance.

Thanks to the Cooper Institute for Aerobics Research, Dallas, Texas, with special thanks to Gregory Welk, Ph.D., former director of the Cooper Institute's Division of Childhood and Adolescent Health. Dr. Welk is now an assistant professor with the Department of Health and Human Performance at Iowa State University. Thanks also to research assistant Donna Fischer. The BSA appreciates their personal involvement with the 1999 revision of this pamphlet.

Photo and Illustration Credits

Jupitermages—cover *(scale);* pages 2–5, 15, 18 *(top),* 61, 65, and 73

Doug Menuez/Sports and Recreation 2/©1999–2005 Getty Images—page 6

©Photos.com—cover *(all except merit badge and scale);* pages 19, 26 *(background),* 27, 30, 37, 40–41 *(both),* and 71

Karl Weatherly/Sports and Recreation 2/©1999–2005 Getty Images—page 74 *(inset)*

U.S. Department of Agriculture, courtesy—page 42

All other photos and illustrations not mentioned above are the property of or are protected by the Boy Scouts of America.

John McDearmon—pages 56 *(illustration)* and 57

Christian Michaels—page 81

Brian Payne—pages 10, 24, 32, and 74 *(top)*

Randy Piland—page 6

Scott Stenjem—page 44